A Guide to Practical Health Promotion

Mary Gottwald and Jane Goodman-Brown

Open University Press

Open University Press
McGraw-Hill Education
McGraw-Hill House
Shoppenhangers Road
Maidenhead
Berkshire
England
SL6 2QL

email: enquiries@openup.co.uk
world wide web: www.openup.co.uk

and Two Penn Plaza, New York, NY 10121-2289, USA

First published 2012

A catalogue record of this book is available from the British Library

ISBN-13: 978–0–33–524459–1 (pb)
ISBN-10: 0–33–524459–9 (pb)
eISBN: 978–0–33–524460–7

Library of Congress Cataloging-in-Publication Data
CIP data applied for

Typesetting and e-book compilations by
RefineCatch Limited, Bungay, Suffolk
Printed in the UK by Bell and Bain Ltd, Glasgow.

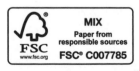

The **McGraw·Hill** Companies

A Guide to Practical
Health Promotion

"This text represents a useful, well-pitched contribution ... The book is densely packed but skilfully written to feel comfortable for the reader; challenging in places but never to the extent to discourage engagement."

Jane Thomas, Acting Head of College of Human and Health Sciences,

Swansea University, UK

Contents

7 The Mass Media and Social Marketing   170
Mary Gottwald and Jane Goodman-Brown

Acknowledgements

The authors would like to thank the following individuals for their help during the writing of this book: Gail Lansdown and Jackie Miley.

Figures

Tables

Overview of the Book

Introduction

This text is aimed at allied health professionals, nurses and practitioners engaged in health promotion, health improvement programmes and those expecting to practise in this area in the future without necessarily having any specific training, with the intention of making links between health promotion theory and practice. It is also intended for use by students studying at either undergraduate or post qualifying undergraduate level.

Our experience of delivering teaching on health promotion, at both post qualifying and postgraduate level, has highlighted that although learners understand the theory they find it challenging to apply the theory to their practice. This text will therefore enable readers to develop their problem solving skills, in order to select appropriate activities to use within practice to empower individuals to make the decision to change their health related behaviours.

We have found that the literature uses different terminology that is synonymous, for example, health promotion, health prevention, health promotion programmes and interventions. In this book we use health promotion and health promotion programmes and interventions as appropriate.

Structure of the book

Each chapter follows the same format. A short introduction will be given which explains the contents and this will be followed by learning objectives. Key points will be identified and activities are included, which will encourage you to reflect on your own practice. Each chapter will discuss health promotion theories and will then apply the theory to four case scenarios. At the end of each chapter key points and implications for practice will be listed and finally some questions will be posed. The suggested answers to these questions are in the Appendix

1

(p. 198). The book is divided into two sections: Part 1 sets the context and Part 2 presents suggestions on how individuals and communities can be empowered.

Chapter 1

This chapter presents the four case scenarios that are applied throughout the book. The main focus of this chapter is to illustrate that the concept of health is not straightforward, and therefore when promoting health and well-being, we need to recognize and understand the various dimensions and determinants of health, and the difference between health inequalities and health inequities. In addition, we have to recognize that health beliefs can also affect an individual's health related decision making, and that an individual's health and well-being can be influenced by a range of factors, both within and outside the individual's control. Policies underpin health promotion programmes, and this chapter introduces a number of World Health Organisation conferences that have led to the development of policies that aim to narrow the health divide and achieve equity within health care.

Chapter 2

This chapter illustrates the breadth of application to health promotion activity and the diversity in which health promotion takes place, for example, schools, prisons, rehabilitation/enablement centres, communities and hospitals. Considering the contexts and ideas will help you to understand a number of aspects for exploration. Therefore, when planning health promotion work with an individual or group of individuals, you will need to think about the situation and then which approach(es) – i.e. educational, behavioural, medical, societal or empowerment – could be applied. You will also need to think about which level of health promotion is appropriate – primary, secondary or tertiary.

Chapter 3

There are a number of models available to us to consider, and this chapter focuses on three. This chapter illustrates how The Stages of Change, Health Belief and Health Action health promotion models can help us to understand how individuals might make the decision to change their health related behaviour. If those engaged in health promotion activity are aware of a number of health promotion models, then they can compare and contrast them, and choose the most appropriate model to guide their decision making for each individual or group of individuals. This chapter also considers motivational interviewing and links this to the Stages of Change Model. Finally this chapter considers how the choice of model also depends on the individual's culture, personal values and beliefs, and socio-economic and environmental status.

Chapter 4

This chapter explores the role of self-awareness in helping individuals to improve their health. Attitudes and behaviours are linked to Rotter's locus of control, and this helps us to understand how people's attitudes towards change affect whether or not they can change. We explore how Antonovsky's theory helps us to understand that values influence the individual's willingness to participate in health enhancing behaviours. In the previous chapter we introduced self-esteem and self-efficacy as part of the Health Action Model and this chapter highlights how these concepts are prerequisites for successful behavioural change. Finally this chapter explains the role that self-confidence and advocacy have in developing self-awareness and how this helps an individual with decision making and changing behaviour.

Chapter 5

This chapter emphasizes that working in partnership with individuals who are considering health related behavioural change is crucial to health promotion work. The aim of health promotion is to empower individuals, and they are less likely to feel empowered if we make health related decisions and set goals for them. Therefore establishing a rapport, being empathetic, communicating clearly and negotiating are basic skills required for health promotion practitioners. Furthermore, in order to facilitate life skills such as assertiveness, communication and problem solving, there are a number of health promotion activities that we need to consider, and this chapter emphasizes that the focus should not solely be on health education, even though it has an important part to play in health promotion work. However, in order for behavioural change to be achieved, this chapter considers *how* we can develop confidence, self-esteem, assertiveness, problem solving and literacy skills.

Chapter 6

This chapter explores the role of groups and group dynamics, including group structure and development and the impact that these have when planning health promotion programmes. Activities within groups are considered and applied to practice using the case scenarios, and it is suggested that interventions are most effective if they are client centred, hands on activities.

The chapter will explore how a community is defined, and the implications of this for health promotion, and discuss why communities have an important role in promoting health. Furthermore, it discusses the concept of social capital and identifies the key characteristics that need to be developed within communities.

Chapter 7

The final chapter examines mass media as an important channel of communication and critiques the strengths and limitations of using mass media approaches. The diffusion of innovation theory, the direct effects/aerosol spray model and the communication-behaviour change model are explored, compared and applied to practice. This chapter ends with an exploration of how social marketing can be used to apply the principles used in marketing to social situations, and focuses on the issues from the perspective of the consumer.

Part 1

Context setting

1

An Introduction to Why Health Promotion is Important

Mary Gottwald and Jane Goodman-Brown

Chapter contents

Introduction

In 1978, the Alma Ata Declaration identified the goal of 'health for all by 2000', and although this has not yet been achieved, it is evident that throughout the world improving health through health promotion is clearly on government agendas, for example, the UK Government White Paper *Healthy Lives, Healthy People* (DH 2010). This chapter explores health, health beliefs, health determinants and health inequalities, and briefly discusses strategic actions taken to improve the health of the population, identified by the World Health Organisation. Four case scenarios are presented, which will be used throughout this book to help you understand how health promotion can empower individuals to make the decision to change their health related behaviour. Policy underpins all health promotion work, however specific policies will not be covered in this book and therefore readers will need to explore policies that relate to their own countries.

Learning objectives

By the end of this chapter the reader will be better able to:

- Discuss the historical perspective and role of the World Health Organisation in international health promotion work
- Identify the dimensions and determinants of health
- Critically evaluate definitions of health
- Explore the concept of inequalities in health, and its role in health promotion
- Differentiate between inequalities and inequity in health care
- Identify and locate local and national policies relating to their own country

The case scenarios

Case scenario 1: Emily

Emily is 6 years old and is reluctant to take exercise; she prefers to watch TV or play on her hand-held computer terminal, and she is choosy about the food she will eat. Her mum, Karen, is a single parent and lives in a rented house in a small town with Emily and her younger brother Josh who is 3 years old. Karen tends to feed them quickly prepared, cheap food which is high in saturated fats and carbohydrates. Karen mainly does this because this is what the children like, but also because it is cheap and her cooking skills are limited.

In Emily's class, many of the children are similar to her in that they dislike physical activity and prefer to play computer games rather than play outside. The class has been doing a project on healthy eating, and the teacher is dismayed by their lack of knowledge about food. She asks the school nurse to become involved, and they design a primary health promotion project on healthy diet and exercise for the children and their families. Part of the project includes cookery demonstrations, which parents are invited to, and free activities at the local sports centre for the whole family.

Furthermore, to raise the children's awareness of their physical fitness, they are all weighed and measured. They plot their measurements on a class chart to identify that they are all different, and to help to develop their self-awareness. Parents are invited to come in and see the results of this exercise. Emily's mum realizes that Emily is one of the heaviest in the class, and she discusses with the school nurse how to reduce her weight. An action plan for Emily is designed by Karen and the school nurse, and Emily's mum asks if Josh can be included in the plan, as she is concerned about his weight too.

Case scenario 2: Hamed

Hamed is a 42-year-old married man who lives in his own house with his family, his wife Halima and two boys aged 10 and 8. He works in the family taxi business, and since taking over the responsibility for promoting the business the annual profits have increased. His hours are long and involve lots of sitting and very little exercise. Hamed enjoys his food, and his wife is a good traditional cook. Recently he has put on quite a lot of weight and he is always thirsty.

Hamed's father was diagnosed with diabetes at the age of 45 and Halima is concerned that Hamed may also have a problem. She notices a poster, at the local surgery, which explains the signs and symptoms of diabetes. It also offers free diabetes screening tests to anyone with a family history of diabetes. She enquires further and is referred to the practice nurse. The practice nurse takes Hamed's details, and makes an appointment for him to come in and see her.

Hamed goes for the appointment, and his blood glucose level indicates that he may have diabetes type II. The nurse gives him written information about improving his diet and increasing exercise, which she goes through with him to ensure he understands. She also offers to see Halima, as Hamed states that Halima does all the cooking and shopping. The nurse also suggests that he might like to attend a support group at the local community centre, that has been set up to help newly diagnosed diabetics cope with the change in lifestyle.

Case scenario 3: Richard

Richard is a 62-year-old deputy head of a large secondary school. He is divorced, having separated from his wife five years ago. He has a son and a daughter, both married and well. However, they do not live nearby and at times this makes Richard feel sad.

Richard has had three admissions to a psychiatric unit for depression, the last admission being a year ago. Recently he presented to the GP with two or three episodes of chest tightness and generally feeling unwell. An ECG was undertaken in the GP surgery, and it showed a degree of ischaemia that needed further investigation. Richard was referred to the Acute Chest Pain clinic at the hospital, and assessed for cardiac disease. At the clinic Richard took a stress test and after five minutes of the protocol was found to have chest ECG changes and to have experienced some chest pain. On angiogram it was found that Richard's two major coronaries were blocked and he required insertion of a coronary stent.

Richard's father died 20 years ago (aged 64) following a myocardial infarction. He has two brothers; one has hypertension and the other, as far as he knows, is fit and well. Richard has never had his cholesterol checked.

Richard has smoked 20 cigarettes a day for 35 years; he does no formal exercise although he does walk to work every day. He admits to drinking approximately 30 units of spirits per week. He lives on his own and often cannot be 'bothered' to cook, so tends to snack. He does not feel overly stressed; however work is very busy and he works long hours with very little relaxation time.

He has had his stent inserted and is on anti-platelets for a minimum of one year, and has been commenced on an ACE inhibitor for his hypertension. His cholesterol result came back as 7.1 so he has also been commenced on statins.

He has been referred to the cardiac rehabilitation team prior to discharge. His main needs are weight control, exercise, diet, smoking and alcohol input, and medicine management.

Case scenario 4: David

David is 27 years old and has served a number of prison terms. Currently he is serving a two year sentence for drug related crimes.

David had difficulty at school and was labelled as having a hyper-activity disorder. He left school at 15, has never been employed and has been homeless on and off when not in prison, but sometimes stays with friends.

David's mother visits when she can, but finds it difficult to afford the fare.

David has a history of drug misuse, and as and when he can, drinks large quantities of cheap alcohol. He continues to take drugs, but has changed his normal substance to avoid detection. He has also smoked cigarettes since he was 11.

David receives health services within the prison system, and is part of a programme to combine health care with rehabilitation and resettlement in the outside world, and to reduce the incidence of re-offending. Recently he attended the medical clinic with a nasty cough and received advice on how the prison quit smoking campaign is particularly success-ful. He has signed up for a smoking cessation group and is beginning to commit to giving up smoking. There are more and more no-smoking areas within the prison and some with good TV.

David notices that the prison is cleaner than the last time he was confined. He attended a clinic where his drug misuse was addressed, and he can now take part in a needle-exchange programme. He has been offered a place on a detox programme and is reassured by the promise of contact with support services when he is released. He has been screened for blood borne viruses and had an immunization for Hepatitis B.

A mental health nurse (from the in-reach team) within the prison meets regularly with David to discuss his learning difficulties, and has organized for him to work in the prison kitchen. He has also been offered a place in a reading class to help him catch up on his lost schooling.

A new programme is being offered by the prison on building respect and understanding. David would like to sign up for this, although places are limited, as he finds life outside the prison a great hardship, and would like to make some changes to his life when his sentence is complete.

Health

Before we consider health promotion theory, it is important that we first consider the concept of health. Defining the concept of health is not straightforward. Due to the different dimensions and determinants of health, a number of definitions have been presented. Definitions of health can be influenced by culture, religious beliefs, age, gender, education and life experiences.

The World Health Organisation (1946) originally defined health as 'a state of complete physical, mental and social well-being and not merely the absence of disease and infirmity'. Although this definition is widely used in the literature, it only really considers that *health is the absence of disease,* and this indicates a medical model. One could also argue against this definition, because those who could be considered 'not in a state of complete physical, mental and social well-being' may well view themselves as healthy; for example, an individual with rheumatoid arthritis who is able to achieve their objectives on a daily basis may not consider themselves unhealthy.

This definition implies that 'health' and 'well-being' mean the same. However, Walker and John (2012) refer back to the ancient Greeks, who defined health (Hygeia) and well-being (eudaimonia/happiness) differently. Health is linked to well-being but tends to have a disease focus, whereas well-being includes the social determinants of health. Well-being can be measured, both subjectively and object-ively, and therefore could be used to evaluate the impact of policies and health promotion programmes (Walker and John 2012).

For some time now the UK Government has promoted the importance of five-a-day fruit and vegetables, to improve health and well-being. The New Economics Foundation (2008, cited in Walker and John 2012: 41) takes this further and suggests that it is important for well-being for individuals to include the following five actions in their daily lives:

- **Connecting with people** For example, children can develop friendships at school, through local organizations such as guides and scouts and through the church. These friendships can support and sustain them throughout life.

- **Being active** Choosing an activity that is enjoyable is crucial and this does not necessarily mean strenuous exercise. Outdoor bowls, walking, gardening, rowing, running and playing golf are just a few examples.

- **Taking notice** Noticing the environment around us, for example, the changing colours of the leaves in the autumn; noticing that it does not get dark so early in the evenings; listening to the sounds of the birds singing; noticing the first lambs in the spring.

- **Continuous learning** Learning can be fun and does not necessarily mean studying to degree level or a qualification. Setting ourselves goals and challenges can increase our self-esteem and confidence, such as learning how to follow and cook a new recipe once a month; learning to swim as an adult; learning the basics of a new language; learning to mend a bicycle puncture.

- **Giving** Giving something to a friend or colleague at work does not need to cost anything and could include offering to help a colleague who feels pressurized. It could involve joining the WI (Women's Institute) and volunteering to help serve coffee and sandwiches in hospitals. Helping others can increase our own happiness and also helps us to make connections and establish friendships with others.

So it would seem that health and well-being are both important concepts for us to consider.

Forty years later the World Health Organisation (WHO 1986) reviewed its first definition of health given above, and this is stated in the Ottawa Charter (WHO 1986: 1):

> To reach a state of complete physical, mental and social well-being, an individual or group must be able to realize aspirations, to satisfy needs, and to change or cope with the environment. Health is therefore seen as a resource for everyday life, not the objective of living. Health is a positive concept, emphasizing social and personal resources, as well as physical capacities.

This definition is more holistic in that in considers the individual's needs. Seedhouse (2001, cited in Whithead and Irvine 2010: 2) views health as being 'equivalent to a set of conditions that enable individuals to achieve their realistic, chosen and biological potential – and recognizes that the importance of these conditions depends on the individual context'.

Lucas and Lloyd (2005: 7) consider a number of definitions, for example 'health is about achieving personal potential'; 'health can be bought by investing in private health care, sold via health food shops, given by drugs or surgery, and lost by accidents or disease'; (Aggleton 1994, cited in Lucas and Lloyd 2005: 7) and 'individuals have a reserve of well-being, individually determined by constitution and temperament as well as a positive state of equilibrium' (Herzlich 1973, cited in Lucas and Lloyd 2005: 7).

What all of these definitions have in common is that although health relates to each individual, the level of health achieved varies depending on beliefs, circumstances and other factors, such as those considered above.

Key points

There are different definitions of health to consider
Individual health depends on a number of factors

Health beliefs, health dimensions and determinants

The World Health Organisation, along with international governments, has consistently worked to improve the health of the population; however, health inequalities continue to exist internationally.

In order to understand why inequalities continue to exist, we need to recognize that health beliefs, dimensions and determinants of health can also affect whether an individual considers themselves to be healthy or not. Health beliefs and personal perceptions can be influenced by gender, age, culture and socio-economic status (Piper 2009). Individual health beliefs can also change during a person's lifetime, due to life experiences, and therefore individual definitions of health may also change. For example, if someone believed that being healthy was the absence of disease, but later develops a chronic disease such as diabetes, they may still feel that they are healthy despite the disease. Therefore their perception of health has changed; if they are able to achieve everything they want, then they may well perceive themselves to be healthy.

As stated in the Jakarta Declaration (WHO 1997: 1), 'health is a basic human right and is essential for social and economic development'. The Ottawa Charter (WHO 1986: 1) states that 'good health is a major resource for social, economic and personal development and an important dimension of quality of life'.

> **Key point**
>
> Health promotion work must consider all of the dimensions of health

Therefore when considering health it is important to reflect on the physical, mental, emotional, social, spiritual and sexual aspects of individuals. It is also crucial to take into account how societal, environmental and global issues influence these dimensions.

Physical health relates to body status, i.e. fitness and absence of disease and illness. **Mental health** concerns the psychological status of the individual; their perceived feelings of value and well-being. For **emotional health** it is important that an individual can both recognize and express their emotions (Naidoo and Wills 2009; Scriven 2010).

Naidoo and Wills (2009) and Scriven (2010) go on to highlight that feeling cared for and loved is also essential, and can affect the ability to make and maintain relationships. Feeling that support is available from friends and family and being able to engage with others leads to **social health** being sustained (Naidoo and Wills 2009; Scriven 2010). In 2005 the World Health Organisation estab-lished the Commission on Social Determinants of Health (CSDH). The remit for the CSDH was to investigate what could be done to promote global health equity. This commission, which reported in 2008, provides advice on how to reduce inequities in particular resulting from social determinants of health.

Three key recommendations were made:

1   Improve daily living conditions

2   Tackle the inequitable distribution of power, money and resources

3   Measure and understand the problems and assess the impact of action.

(WHO 2008: 6)

For **spiritual health** it is important to be able to recognize, express and practise one's own core beliefs, i.e. religious views, morals and values. It is also important for an individual to recognize, express and practise their own sexual preferences for sexual health (Naidoo and Wills 2009; Scriven 2010).

As well as the above dimensions, there are wider determinants (societal and global) that could impact on whether an individual is healthy or not. In a society where the infrastructure is inadequate to the extent that basic shelter, clean water, food and income are limited, and where basic human rights may also be restricted, then health could be affected. The third international conference at Sundsvall (1991) identified that women, the majority of the world's population, are oppressed and discriminated against in the labour market and to some extent today this remains the case (Naidoo and Wills 2009; Scriven 2010).

> **Key point**
>
> Health promotion work must also consider these wider dimensions of health

Over the last few years a number of countries (Haiti, China, Japan, Australia, New Zealand and USA) have experienced severe floods, cyclones, earthquakes and tsunamis. Individuals have lost their homes; children have lost access to educa-tion; sanitation has been affected, leading to outbreaks of cholera in some areas; and all of these have an impact on health. Lastly, according to Naidoo and Wills (2009: 4), 'caring for the planet and ensuring its sustainability for the future' is vital.

Health is also dependent on a number of dynamic interactions of different variables, and the health and well-being of individuals is influenced by a range of factors, both within and outside the individual's control. These factors are often known as determinants of health.

Figure 1.1 illustrates a number of aspects that could affect the health of individuals and is based on Dahlgren and Whitehead's (1991) model. The age, gender and hereditary factors in the main are fixed; individuals may like to deny they are getting older, however, the fact is that each year we all become another year older. Individuals are able to express their sexuality, and in some cases due to technological advances, undergo surgery to change gender; however, as already said, age, gender and hereditary factors in the main do not change.

Dahlgren and Whitehead's (1991) model will now be illustrated using the example of smoking.

Applying this model: smoking

Initially individuals may choose whether to smoke or not, however, smoking is addictive. There are also **social and community influences** that may affect the decision to begin smoking or to stop smoking, for example, peer pressure and family norms. If an individual's friends and family smoke, then they may feel

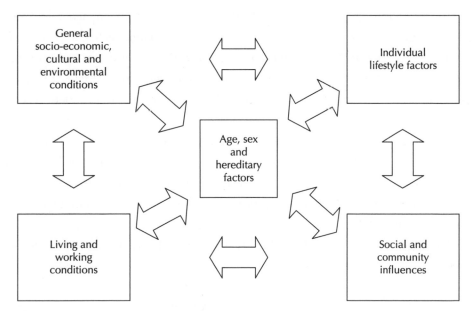

Figure 1.1 The main determinants of health
Source: Adapted from Dahlgren and Whitehead (1991)

pressurized to smoke. **Living conditions and unemployment** could be factors in determining whether an individual makes the decision to smoke or not. Living in poor housing where amenities are limited can cause depression and stress as can unemployment, and so smoking can relieve this stress and reduce anxiety momentarily. Poor **environmental conditions** such as pollution can also cause stress and anxiety so individuals may choose to smoke to relieve these emotional feelings. **General socio-economic, cultural and environmental conditions** might influence the decision to smoke, such as the cost and accessibility of cigarettes.

Activity

- Reflect on some of the individuals you work with and think of a different example to smoking.
- Apply Dahlgren and Whitehead's (1991) model.

Health inequalities

In this section inequalities are defined, the difference between health inequalities and health inequity is explained, and the links to health promotion practice are explored.

The determinants of health were discussed in the previous section and this helped us to see that health is complex and is influenced by a variety of factors. Understanding the complexity of health will help to develop your understanding of health inequalities.

Definitions of health inequalities vary in different countries and have changed over time. In the UK, health inequalities are debated but are acknowledged as important (DH 2010). In the USA the term is not used; instead there is discussion of health disparities, which makes comparisons between different countries difficult (Graham 2007).

It is suggested (Graham 2007) that there are three different meanings to health inequalities:

1 differences between the health of individuals;
2 differences between the health of populations;

3   differences between those occupying unequal positions in the social hierarchy.

In health promotion, it is generally the differences in health status between different populations, and those as a result of social hierarchies, that are of concern. The differences can be between those who have limited economic and social resources compared to those with greater economic and social resources, and this is often seen as being linked to social class (Scriven 2010). This gap between rich and poor is reported to be widening in many societies (Scriven 2010). However, Davies and Macdowall (2006) propose that it is not just social class that has an impact on health, but also geography, age, gender, disability and ethnicity. These factors can also cause health inequalities.

Examination of the health differences between groups demonstrates that health follows a social pattern. An example might be examining perceived differences in health status linked to household income. Those in the lowest quintile of incomes tend to have a more negative view of their health (40 per cent reporting their health is not good), as opposed to those in the highest quintile, where only 15 per cent report their health is not good (Graham 2007). This reflects that those in low income groups tend to have poorer health.

Looking at health in relation to social hierarchies suggests that it is those from socially disadvantaged groups – whether as a result of finance or position in society, for example, ethnic groups – who are more likely to have poor health than those from advantaged groups. This suggests that inequalities in health are linked to social inequalities, rather than just being the result of general health (Graham 2007). Green and Tones (2010) suggest that inequalities are the result of unequal opportunities in health, which lead to further social inequalities.

Since the 1970s and the Black Report (Townsend et al. 1992), there has been an increasing interest in inequalities and the causes of them. Reports by the UK Labour government during their period in office support the breadth of inequalities, indicating that inequalities are due to the interaction of a range of factors and cannot be ascribed to any one area (Hubley and Copeman 2008). The current government has indicated that they intend to continue to try and address inequalities (DH 2010). This continuation is important as comparison between countries shows that it is not the richest societies that have the best health, but those that have the smallest difference in income between rich and poor, leading to an egalitarian society with equal opportunities which results in better health overall (Ewles and Simnett 2003).

Graham (2007) suggests that heath inequalities are descriptive, and although they help to explain patterns of health, they do not address the whole issue of difference. Health inequity, in contrast, refers to different opportunities for health for populations. Inequities may be as a result of unequal access to resources such as nutritious food, housing or health services. Regardless of the cause, health inequities are differences in health which are considered to be unfair and unjust (Whitehead 1990, cited in Graham 2007).

> **Key point**
>
> Health inequity refers to different opportunities for health

Differences between individuals and groups at different points in their lives are to be expected; for example individuals are often healthier when they are young rather than older. This can also be seen in groups, i.e. younger people as a group tend to be healthier than older people. Nevertheless differences in health as a result of social hierarchies can be considered as examples of health inequity: if an individual is unhealthy because they are unemployed and cannot afford healthy food, this is inequity because their lack of healthy food is the result of their position in society, rather than any choices they may have made. The same is true of groups of people. For example, if those from an identified ethnic group live in poor housing through their inability to afford better quality housing rather than through choice, this in an inequity which will have an impact on their health. Health inequity links to moral debates about what is fair and just in society, so it tends to be a complex matter.

As health promoters it is essential that there is an understanding of the health of populations, and how this is influenced by a range of factors often beyond individual control to enable the planning of appropriate interventions (Green and Tones 2010). Health promotion is criticized for focusing on individual behaviour change, which does not recognize the range of influences on health that have been discussed, and as a result does not address inequalities (Hubley and Copeman 2008). Scriven (2010) suggests that health promotion activities might only reach those with the resources to address their health issues, thus widening inequalities, therefore it is essential that we as health promoters have an in-depth understanding of inequalities in health.

Activity

- From your practice, identify a health inequality.
- Now try to identify a health inequity.

The role of the World Health Organisation in supporting health promotion

As mentioned above, a number of international conferences have helped to develop our understanding of health promotion strategies, and have placed 'health for all' and health promotion firmly on the agenda. Policies have been developed from these conferences in order to narrow the health divide in society and ensure equity within health care, thus reducing the inequalities within deprived and vulnerable groups.

Activity

- Identify some national policies linked to improving the health of the population.
- What is the key aim of each policy?
- What are the key objectives?
- Is an action plan identified? If so, make a note of strategies suggested.

Representatives from developed countries attending these conferences helped to develop policies that would impact positively on developing countries. Delegates from 42 countries participated in the Adelaide conference of 1977, and by the time the Nairobi conference was held in 2009, over one hundred countries engaged in discussions. Table 1.1 summarizes key points from each conference held to date.

Table 1.1   World Health Organisation conferences

1978 Alma Ata Declaration	Key target: an acceptable level of health for all by the year 2000. Emphasized the role of health education, developing and implementing primary health care and the need to reduce health inequalities. (WHO 1978)
1986 The Ottawa Charter	Built on the Alma Ata declaration. Focused on the key functions of strategies, advocacy, enabling and mediation. Emphasized five action areas for health promotion:

1 Building healthy public policy
2 Creating supportive environments
3 Strengthening community action
4 Developing personal skills
5 Re-orientating health services
(WHO 1986)

1988 Adelaide Charter	Emphasized health as a fundamental social goal, which could only be achieved with the development of public policy and public participation and cooperation between all sectors of society. Emphasized healthy public policy needed to 'ensure that advances in health-care technology help, rather than hinder, the process of achieving improvements in equity'. (WHO 1988: 7)
1991 Sundsvall conference	Emphasized the need to develop supportive environments, i.e. the social dimension, the political dimension, the economic dimension and the need to use women's skills and knowledge in all sectors. Focused on the importance of action to achieve social justice. (WHO 1991)
1997 Jakarta Declaration	The first conference to be held in a developing country, and the first to involve the private sector in supporting health promotion. This conference focused on health promotion into the twenty-first century and emphasized the need to promote social responsibility; to involve families and communities in health promotion activities; to develop partnerships with the private sector; to develop the infrastructure for health promotion; to empower individuals and increase investment in health. (WHO 1997)
2000 Mexico City global conference	Emphasized that in order to achieve 'health for all' and 'equity in health' in the twenty-first century, health promotion must be an essential component of public policies and health promotion programmes internationally. (WHO 2000)

| 2005 | Bangkok Charter | Reviewed health promotion strategies internationally and identified the need for 'coherent policies, investment and partnership across governments, international organizations, civil society and the private sector to ensure that health promotion is central to the global development agenda'. (WHO 2005: 1) |
| 2009 | The Nairobi global conference | Adoption of Nairobi Call for Action and identified 'key strategies to reduce the implementation gap in health and development through health promotion'. Focused on practical issues in 'building empowered communities; identified strategic actions required to achieve health literacy and practical linkages between health promotion and health care systems'. (WHO 2009: 1) |

Common themes

There are a number of common themes from these conferences. Each conference identifies the importance of health promotion work and that the focus of health promotion should be on equity, enablement, empowerment and community action. Each also identifies that policy should avoid harming the health of the individual; protect the environment; restrict the production of, and trade in, potentially harmful goods such as tobacco; safeguard both the citizen in the marketplace and the individual in the workplace; and include equity-focused health impact assessments as an integral part of policy development (Jakarta Declaration, cited in Green and Tones 2010).

> **Key point**
>
> Policy underpins all health promotion work

Chapter summary

In this chapter we have illustrated that the concept of health is not straight-forward, and therefore when promoting health and well-being, we need to recognize and understand the various dimensions and determinants of health and recognize the difference between health inequalities and health inequities. In addition we have to recognize that health beliefs can also affect an individual's health-related decision making, and that the health and well-being of individuals can be influenced by a range of factors, both within and outside the individual's control. This chapter has also introduced a number of World Health Organisation conferences that have led to the development of policies that aim to narrow the health divide and achieve equity within health care.

Key points

- Health is multidimensional and can be influenced by culture, religious beliefs, age, gender, education and life experience.

- It is important for those working within health promotion to consider the dimensions and determinants of health.

- Inequalities in health persist, and as health promoters, it is vital that we understand why they occur and address them through our work.

- The World Health Organisation is committed to improving the health of the population, and is active in pursuing this aim.

- Governments in all countries are stewards of the health of their nation.

Implications for practice

- Practitioners need to understand that there are many factors that impact on health.

- Practitioners need to acknowledge that inequalities continue to be an issue that needs to be addressed through health promotion.

- Improving health and well-being involves individuals as well health and social care professionals and international organizations such as the World Health Organisation.

End of chapter questions

1 How does an understanding of health and its determinants impact on your practice?

2 What is the difference between health inequality and health inequity?

3 What is the role of the World Health Organisation in promoting health and well-being?

References

Dahlgren, G. and Whitehead, M. (1991) *Policies and Strategies to Promote Equity in Health*. Stockholm: Institute for Future Studies.

Davies, M. and Macdowall, W. (2006) *Health Promotion Theory*. Maidenhead: Open University Press.

DH (Department of Health) (2010) *Healthy Lives, Healthy People*. London: HMSO.

Ewles, L. and Simnett, I. (2003) *Promoting Health: A Practical Guide*, 5th edn. Edinburgh: Ballière Tindall.

Graham, H. (2007) *Unequal Lives: Health and Socioeconomic Inequalities*. Maidenhead: Open University Press.

Green, J. and Tones, K. (2010) *Health Promotion: Planning and Strategies*. London: Sage.

Hubley, J. and Copeman, J. (2008) *Practical Health Promotion*. Cambridge: Polity.

Lucas, K. and Lloyd, B. (2005) *Health Promotion: Evidence and Experience*. London: Sage.

Naidoo, J. and Wills, J. (2009) *Foundations for Health Promotion*. London: Baillière Tindall Elsevier.

Piper, S. (2009) *Health Promotion for Nurses: Theory and Practice*. London and New York: Routledge.

Scriven, A. (2010) *Promoting Health: A Practical Guide*. London: Baillière Tindall Elsevier.

Townsend, P., Davidson, N. and Whitehead, M. (1992) *Inequalities in Health: The Black Report and the Health Divide*. London: Penguin.

Walker, P. and John, M. (2012) *From Public Health to Wellbeing*. Basingstoke: Palgrave Macmillan.

WHO (World Health Organisation) (1946) *Constitution of the World Health Organisation*. www.who.int/governance/eb/who-constitution-en.pdf (accessed 29 November 2011).

WHO (1978) *Alma Ata Declaration*. http://www.euro.who.int/en/who-we-are/policy-documents/declaration-of-alma-ata (accessed 25 October 2010).

WHO (1986) *The Ottawa Charter*. http://www.who.int/healthpromotion/conferneces/previous/ottawa/en. (accessed 25 October 2010).

WHO (1988) *The Adelaide Charter*. http://www.who.int/healthpromotion/conferneces/previous/adelaide/en (accessed 25 October 2010).

WHO (1991) *The Sundsvall Conference*. http://www.who.int/healthpromotion/conferneces/previous/sundsvall/en (accessed 25 October 2010).

WHO (1997) *The Jakarta Declaration*. http://www.who.int/healthpromotion/conferneces/previous/jakarta/en (accessed 25 October 2010).

WHO (2000) *Mexico City Global Conference*. http://www.who.int/healthpromotion/conferneces/previous/jakarta/en (accessed 25 October 2010).

WHO (2005) *The Bangkok Charter*. http://www.who.int/mediacentre/news/releases/2005/pr34/en/ (accessed 25 October 2010).

WHO (2009) *The Nairobi Conference*. http://www.who.int/healthpromotion/conferences/7gchp/en/ (accessed 25 October 2010).

WHO (2008) *Closing the Gap in a Generation: Health Equity* Through Action on the Social Determinants of Health. http://whqlibdoc.who.int/hq/2008/WHO_IER_CSDH_08.1_eng.pdf (accessed 7 November 2010).

2

An Overview of Health Promotion Theory
Mary Gottwald and Jane Goodman-Brown

Chapter contents

Introduction

This chapter will provide an overview of some aspects of health promotion theory. There are numerous books that discuss health promotion theory in detail, and references will be provided that will facilitate your understanding in more depth. The focus of this book is on the application of health promotion theory and not the theory per se, however, it is important that we sketch out the key theories before applying them to the case scenarios, so you are aware of the different concepts.

First of all a number of definitions of health promotion will be considered. Those engaged within health promotion work will be working in a variety of contexts, and therefore this chapter will consider the levels and approaches to health promotion work that can be used within these different contexts. As we go through this chapter, we will use the case scenarios provided in Chapter 1, in order to illustrate the theory discussed.

Learning objectives

By the end of this chapter the reader will be better able to:

- Define and critique definitions of health promotion
- Identify contexts for health promotion work
- Identify key aspects of health promotion work within different contexts
- Identify and apply relevant health promotion approaches to practice
- Recognize appropriate levels of health promotion activity

Definitions of health promotion and the importance of health promotion work

The terms 'health promotion' and 'health education' are sometimes used inter-changeably, however, there is a difference between these two concepts. Although health education is very much part of health promotion, health education is only one aspect of health promotion work. Health education raises awareness and provides individuals with information on why it is important to improve their health, and how individuals can begin to change their health-related behaviours. Health promotion also includes preventative work such as screening for breast cancer and children's immunization programmes. It involves organizational activities that demonstrate consideration to the health of employees, for example, providing healthy options in canteens or access to free gyms. It involves environmental health measures, such as the smoking ban that has been implemented in

Key point

Health promotion includes activities other than health education

numerous countries. It also involves policy making; for example, in order for schools to promote healthy eating, policy directives will have to be provided that enable schools to action healthy eating initiatives throughout the curriculum (Peixoto 2010; Scriven 2010).

Chapter 1 identified a number of international conferences, demonstrating how the World Health Organisation has become an advocate of health promotion, and how health promotion is key to government strategic development. These conferences underpin the importance of health promotion work. To begin with, the Ottawa Charter (WHO 1986: 1) defined health promotion as:

> The process of enabling people to increase control over and to improve their health. To reach a state of complete physical, mental and social well-being, an individual or group must be able to identify and to realize aspirations, to satisfy needs, and to change or cope with the environment.
>
> Health promotion represents a comprehensive social and political process; it not only embraces actions directed at strengthening the skills and capabilities of individuals, but also action directed towards changing social, environmental and economic conditions so as to alleviate their impact on public and individual health. Health promotion is the process of enabling people to increase control over the determinants of health and thereby improve their health. Participation is essential to sustain health promotion action.

This definition highlights that health promotion involves a number of aspects, and responsibility does not just lie with the individual; health promotion needs to be seen as a partnership between the individual, health and social care professionals and policy makers. This is further supported by Naidoo and Wills (2009: 62) who state that 'Health promotion may involve lobbying and political advocacy, but it may just as easily involve working with individuals and groups to enhance their knowledge and understanding of the factors affecting health.'

For this partnership to be successful, it is essential that health promoters involve individuals and groups in all decision making, as this will facilitate empowerment within individuals and groups, who can then decide to continue with their health-related behaviour or

Key points

Health promotion is a partnership between the individual, health and social care professionals and policy makers

The individual must want to change

to change it. Health promotion should not be seen as coercion, but as empowering individuals, and those engaged in health promotion work need to remember that changing behaviour can be difficult. Change also takes time, and we need to make sure that we provide support and guidance in developing skills and strategies that lead to successful behavioural change. However, first of all the individual needs to *want* to change their health-related behaviour.

To sum up the definitions of health promotion, the following is a nice and succinct definition: 'making the healthier choice the easier choice' (Milio 1986, cited in Naidoo and Wills 2000: 84).

Approaches to health promotion

In this section the different approaches that attempt to explain health promotion will be explored, highlighting the advantages and disadvantages of each. They will also be applied to practice. This will be followed by an explanation of the different levels of health promotion (primary, secondary and tertiary) with examples and application to practice.

Health promotion is a complex subject to understand and link to practice; this is highlighted by the variety of approaches to it. Scriven (2010) suggests that there are five different ways of approaching health promotion and that understanding these will help to determine the aims of health promotion. The five approaches are outlined below, along with their advantages and disadvantages.

Medical approach

Focus: the treatment of health conditions in order to promote health or prevent an illness.

Example: immunization.

Advantage of this approach: it is easily measurable, e.g. immunization prevents illness.

Disadvantage of this approach: it does not recognize the wider determinants of health that we discussed in Chapter 1, and assumes that health is the absence of disease (Scriven 2010).

Behaviour change approach

Focus: encourages people to change their behaviour in order to encourage good health.

Example: smoking cessation programme, which urges participants to stop smoking.

Advantage of this approach: initially it would appear to be easy to measure success.

Disadvantages of this approach: it can be difficult to prove that there is a link between the intervention and any subsequent change. A further disadvantage is it is dependent on health and social care experts to support the behaviour change (Naidoo and Wills 2009).

Educational approach

Focus: emphasizes the role of education to develop an individual's knowledge, in order to enable them to change their attitudes and behaviour in relation to their health.

Example: an education programme that does not focus on the need to stop smoking, but is aimed at raising awareness about the benefits of not smoking.

Advantage of this approach: enables individuals to develop their knowledge and change their attitudes.

Disadvantage of this approach: it is time consuming and individuals may not make healthy choices (Naidoo and Wills 2009).

The educational approach differs from a behaviour change approach, in that it does not urge the participants to act in a particular way but helps them to make an informed decision and supports them in their choices. The educational approach suggests that information alone will not necessarily lead to change; a change in attitude is also important.

Client-centred/empowerment approach

Focus: this differs from all of the others, in that it focuses on the individual's perspective, helping them to identify their own health issues and then enabling them to address them. This can take place on an individual basis or in a community.

Example: an example might be discussing their health with an individual who is overweight and finding that they do not want to address their diet, rather they want to address their exercise habits.

Advantage of this approach: It sees Issues from a client's perspective and lets them take the lead.

Disadvantage of this approach: changing behaviour is time consuming (Naidoo and Wills 2009).

Health promoters may not have the skills to help someone become empowered, as this is a gradual process and time consuming. Empowerment can be viewed as one end of a continuum, with coercion at the opposite end and persuasion in the middle (Hubley and Copeman 2008). Empowerment focuses on helping individuals and communities to develop their skills and knowledge and improve their confidence, rather than forcing them to take action or trying to persuade them to change. We will discuss empowerment further in the next chapter, and will link it to activities that could be used with two of the case scenarios.

Similarly an empowerment approach can be used with a community, by helping communities to identify what the important health issues are for them, rather than imposing professionals' predetermined views. This approach helps us to understand that clients and communities have skills and knowledge in relation to health, which should be valued and utilized in order to improve health according to their priorities (Scriven 2010). An example of this could relate to an increase in the number of overweight children in the community. The health promoter may want to focus on increasing the amount of exercise young children engage in within the community; however, the issue for the community might be lack of access to safe play areas.

Social change approach

Focus: focuses on society and how it can change in order to facilitate health.

Example: an example might be the smoking ban in the UK from 2007.

Advantage of this approach: it addresses social issues and generally involves public consultation.

Disadvantage of this approach: it is a top-down approach, and again health promoters may lack the skills to facilitate this kind of approach (Naidoo and Wills 2009).

Deciding which approach to use

In reality most health promotion activities would use more than one approach. For example, a project to encourage physical activity in small children in a deprived area might use an educational approach, to help parents understand the need for regular exercise. It might also use a social change approach through providing facilities for the young children to play. It might also use an empowerment approach by listening to parents' needs and identifying that not only are facilities necessary but support is also required.

> **Key point**
>
> There are strengths and limitations of each approach

Activity

We have explored one model that identifies five different approaches to be considered in health promotion.

- Think of someone that you work with who has a health issue and consider which of these approaches would be most relevant.
- Once you have made your decision ask yourself 'why?'
- This will help you justify your reasons for choices that you make in practice.

From these approaches, it is important to recognize that approaches vary, and will impact on the health promotion activities that we will explore in depth in the following two chapters.

Types of health promotion

Discussing the approaches to health promotion leads us on to consider the different levels of health promotion. Some health promotion is **primary prevention** and aims to prevent ill health, for example, healthy eating education in schools, which would prevent obesity and associated health problems in later life, or parenting programmes for new parents to help develop parenting skills.

Secondary heath promotion aims to help individuals address existing health problems. So, taking the example of eating again, this might be running a healthy eating programme at a GP surgery for adults who are overweight, to help them address the issue. Another example might include a smoking cessation programme for people who have had a heart attack, as this will aim to reduce the likelihood of having another heart attack.

Finally **tertiary health promotion** involves working with people who have an existing condition that cannot be cured, for example, helping people with diabetes to manage their diet through education and skills development, in order to control their diabetes and enable them to prevent further complications. A programme like this might take place in a hospital clinic.

Another example could include an exercise programme for someone with hypertension. This, along with medication, would help the individual to maintain their level of heart health, i.e. blood pressure, within an acceptable range.

Stop and think

The levels of health promotion from a practitioner's perspective are important in helping define what the aim or objective of an intervention might be. The level can also be used to help determine an appropriate setting as indicated in the examples above.

Application of the approaches and levels to the case scenarios

Case scenario 1: Emily

Health promotion in relation to Emily demonstrates a **behaviour change approach,** in that the focus is on helping Emily and her mother to make the decision to change her diet in a specific way. There are also elements of a **social change approach,** as measurement is linked to national policy. Weighing is a form of screening, so this links to a **medical approach,** as the idea is to detect children who have a propensity to be overweight and to address the issue as soon as possible.

This is at a **primary level** because the health promotion activity considers all children within the school. It is also **secondary health promotion** because Emily's BMI is above the normal range and she is overweight.

Case scenario 2: Hamed

This case study uses an **educational approach,** as the information is given, and it is up to Hamed and Halima to choose what they do. A **medical approach** is also used as he was screened for diabetes.

This is **tertiary health promotion,** as Hamed already has an identified condition that cannot be cured. However, the complications can be reduced.

Case scenario 3: Richard

A **behaviour change** and **medical approach** has been used with Richard. He has been screened and he is being encouraged to change his behaviour. A **client-centred approach** has also been used, as Richard has identified a problem by going to see his GP.

Secondary and tertiary health promotion are used in this situation as Richard has an identifiable problem (secondary level) and he will be supported to achieve his full health potential (tertiary level).

Case scenario 4: David

Both **empowerment** and the **educational approach** have been used with David. He has identified that he has issues that need addressing, and he has been supported in achieving change. He has been given information, and how he chooses to behave has been acknowledged, rather than encouraging him to behave in a predetermined way which would be **behaviour** change.

Secondary health promotion is the focus here as he is a smoker and drug user, and he is being helped to address these issues.

Context setting

As well as working on a one-to-one basis and with groups, those engaged in health promotion work could be working in various settings (see Figure 2.1).

Schools

Case scenario 1: Emily

The school nurse and teachers can be involved with not only developing Emily and her class mates' academic abilities, but also supporting their understanding of healthy lifestyles and developing their confidence, self-esteem, social skills and resilience to enable them to make healthy choices.

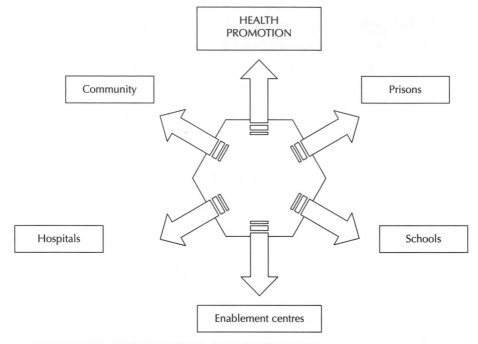

Figure 2.1 Health promotion settings

Schools can provide opportunities to promote health and well-being to children and their families through engaging children in curriculum activities. However, there can be conflict between what the curriculum delivers and what the school canteens and vending machines provide (Rana and Alvaro 2010). Hubley and Copeman (2008) identify three areas where schools can promote health:

1   the school environment

2   school health services

3   health education

Taking these three points into consideration, children eating school meals depend on the skills of the cooks to provide a balanced and nutritional diet, and also the cleanliness of the kitchen environment. They are dependent on learning and playing in safe environments. School nurses working in secondary schools can be involved with promoting well-being through immunization programmes. They could also be involved with reducing the incidence of teenage pregnancies through promoting sexual health and through the dissemination of educational information on alcohol and drugs. In UK primary schools, it is the responsibility of teachers to promote sexual health through the personal, social and health education programmes (PSHE) (Hubley and Copeman 2008).

However, in order to promote children's health and well-being, health promotion workshops could also be provided for all parents and staff, such as on food safety, healthy eating guidelines and planning healthy eating menus. A range of tools could be provided, for example, it may be necessary to carry out a survey on foods provided within schools. Providing a questionnaire, and engaging pupils in gathering this data can motivate them as well as develop their knowledge and understanding. Fact sheets for families, such as nutrition guidelines and what healthy lunch boxes should include could also be provided.

Support for schools from the UK Department of Health (2002)

The Department of Health (2002) provides information and schemes to support schools, for example the school fruit and vegetable scheme, in which all children from 4 to 6 years are provided with a piece of fruit each day.

The National Healthy Schools Programme, which is a joint initiative between the UK Department of Health and Department for Children, Schools and Families (DCSF), has been in place since 1999. In order to gain national recognition for National Healthy Status, schools have had to demonstrate how they are meeting a number of criteria within the curriculum as well as through PSHE. The number of schools achieving this status and having a certificate of recognition has grown over the years, and this can only be beneficial to schools engaged in the Office for Standards in Education (Ofsted) Children's Services and Skills process. Schools now have a healthy schools policy, which states that children are only allowed to bring water to school; vending machines no longer sell chocolate and crisps and school dinners are healthier.

Another government initiative, Change4Life – Eat Well, Move More, Live Longer, is England's first national social marketing campaign, which provides information on eating well and doing more exercise in order to reduce obesity and prolong life. A planning template can be accessed that facilitates the development of a healthy schools approach, and information is provided that assists in the selection of activities. Posters, leaflets, wall charts and activity sheets can be also be downloaded and used within schools (DH 2009).

Other countries have developed similar programmes such as the Health Promoting Schools (HPS) framework in Australia (Rana and Alvaro 2010) and the EatSmart Schools (DH 2006) and EatSmart Restaurant campaigns in Hong Kong (DH 2008). The World Heath Organisation also suggests six key areas for schools to work towards:

In order to improve health, schools can work towards six key areas:

1   school health policies

2   the physical environment of the school

3   the school's social environment

4   community relationships

5   personal health skills

6   school health services

(WHO 1996, cited in Lee et al. 2007: 753)

You can download the latest UK Healthy Schools Toolkit from the Department for Education website. This toolkit provides schools with information on how to carry out a needs assessment, and helps schools to plan, implement and evaluate health promotion initiatives (Department for Education 2011).

Activity

It is useful to make comparisons and get ideas from other resources, so you could compare the information provided in the UK Healthy Schools Toolkit by downloading information from the following links. The EatSmart campaigns in Hong Kong also provide information on suggested healthy menus:

http://www.ahpsa.org.au   (Australian   Health   Promoting   Schools Association) http://www.EatSmart@School.hk (Hong Kong)

http://www.scotland.gov.uk/Topics/Education/Schools/HLivi/foodnutrition (The Schools (Health Promotion and Nutrition) Scotland Act 2007)

If children develop an understanding of healthy lifestyles at an early age, then this can prevent complications such as obesity, drug and alcohol abuse and diabetes type II arising later on. In primary schools cross-curricular links are essential, so the National Curriculum (UK) integrates learning in relation to healthy lifestyles through a number of subjects such as literacy and numeracy, science, art and design and technology. The focus of these activities must not just be on health education, because this alone would only have superficial effects (Peixoto 2010).

We can use the example of a simple activity, such as preparing a fruit salad, to identify how the National Curriculum can help Emily's class to understand the importance of healthy eating.

Application to practice

Case scenario 1: Emily

Class activity: Preparing a fruit salad

Design and technology

- First of all Emily and her class mates can learn about the importance of hand washing and washing the fruit, in order to prevent infections.

- They can learn about the safety of knives.

- In order to prepare a fruit salad they would need to decide which fruit to include; this could be based on colour, taste, texture or nutritional value.

Literacy

- The lessons could focus on developing Emily's language to describe these aspects, for example Emily and her friends could explore what 'sharp' means, as this could link to the knives that are being used, as well the taste of some of the fruit.

- The class would have the opportunity to develop their skills by writing out the instructions on how to make a fruit salad.

Numeracy

- Emily and her class mates could be asked to complete a diary over a week and record their diet.

- Lessons could include children sorting the data into food groups; classifying the food; estimating the number of portions that would be needed for their family.

- Finally Emily could develop her skills by inputting this data into the computer.

- Emily and her class mates could also be given a budget, and could practise their budgeting skills through playing at shops.

- They could be asked to research the cost of fruit, and record this on a spreadsheet to ensure they remain within budget.

Art and design

- Emily and her class could then link their learning to colour, drawing and proportions through designing a poster on how eating fruit is healthy.

- This would encourage creativity, as well as helping the children to understand the messages that posters can deliver.

PSHE

- During PSHE, Emily and her class could set individual goals that would encourage them to lead a healthier lifestyle by eating more fruit, for example: 'By the end of this term I will be eating five portions of fruit and vegetables, three times a week'.

- Teachers can engage Emily's class in a number of activities; for example, they can learn about themselves as individuals; develop skills on how to remain healthy; and develop social skills such as how to resist bullying and teasing if they are overweight.

- The children can learn how to make informed choices, develop a sense of social justice and moral responsibility

Communication is also an essential component of learning; Emily and her class will need to develop planning, communication and decision making skills which are all needed for this simple activity. On completion of this activity, they can also develop evaluation skills and think about their decision making – what went well and what did not work. Chapters 4 and 5 will discuss in more depth how these skills could be encouraged and developed.

Activity

Using the example of exercise answer the following:

- How could the National Curriculum incorporate the importance of exercise?

- Which subjects could include exercise?

- What activities could be used to facilitate primary school children's understanding of exercise?

Prisons

Various individuals can be involved in health promotion work within prisons, for example, educators, nurses, doctors, occupational therapists and prison officers, outside agencies and 'peer education groups' established within prisons (DH 2002).

According to the Department of Health (2002), 80 per cent of prisoners smoke, 24 per cent abuse drugs and 90 per cent experience mental health issues or substance misuse or both.

Prison staff have a duty of care to address the physical, social, mental and environmental health needs of the prison population; prisoners are entitled to the same care as provided by public health care services (DH 2002; Naidoo and Wills 2009). The Social Exclusion Unit (2002: 6) has identified nine key factors that can lead to re-offending: 'lack of education, unemployment, drug and alcohol abuse, poor mental and physical health, poor attitudes and self-control, institutionalisation and lack of life skills, poor housing, lack of financial support and debt and lack of family networks'.

According to the Social Exclusion Report (Social Exclusion Unit 2002: 6):

Many prisoners have experienced a lifetime of social exclusion. Compared with the general population, prisoners are thirteen times as likely to have been in care as a child, thirteen times as likely to be unemployed, ten times as likely to have been a regular truant, two and a half times as likely to have had a family member convicted of a criminal offence, six times as likely to have been a young father and fifteen times as likely to be HIV positive.

Many prisoners' basic skills are very poor. Eighty per cent have the writing skills, 65 per cent the numeracy skills and 50 per cent the reading skills at or below the level of an 11-year-old child. Sixty to 70 per cent of prisoners were using drugs before imprisonment. Over 70 per cent suffer from at least two mental disorders, and 20 per cent of male and 37 per cent of female sentenced prisoners have attempted suicide in the past. The position is often even worse for 18- to 20-year-olds, whose basic skills, unemployment rate and school exclusion background are all over a third worse than those of older prisoners. Health promotion initiatives provide opportunities to address inequalities, as well as the impact of determinants as discussed in Chapter 1. Due to the need to enforce security, individuals may experience loss of autonomy, which can lead to loss of self-esteem; they may experience social exclusion and bullying. *Health Promoting Prisons: A Shared Approach* (DH 2002) outlines strategies for implementing health promotion programmes that enable individuals to adopt healthy behaviours and continue these on release back into the community. There is also a Health in Prisons Project (HIPP) network across Europe, launched by the World Health Organisation in 1995. Initially eight EU countries participated in network meetings but within ten years this had grown to 28. These networking meetings not only highlight current issues and developments related to the health of prisoners, but also include key experts who facilitate the agreement of priorities. Examples of health promotion initiatives to promote behavioural change in those with mental health issues, those who abuse drugs and smokers are considered along with the special needs of minority groups and youths in custody (Gatherer et al. 2005).

Health promotion activities will be explored in depth in Chapters 4 and 5; however, the following are examples of types of health promotion activities that take place in prison settings:

- Prisoners are engaged in producing leaflets or magazines covering aspects such as self-examination and sexual health issues. If collaboration between prison staff and the prisoners is evident, and if prisoners are engaged and their viewpoints valued, then there is more likely to be a change in health-related behaviour.

- Cognitive behavioural skills training can be used to help individuals think about situations, their thoughts, feelings and actions. This helps them to focus on the present, and to make decisions in relation to their health-related behaviour.

- Anger management could be included in a health promotion programme to help with developing calming strategies. These in turn would raise self-esteem, assertiveness and reduce low mood.

- Social and life skills activities could be included, for example, to help with developing assertiveness skills in order to resist peer pressure (for example, to help individuals say 'no' to smoking but 'yes' to using a condom).

- Development of self esteem is important in order to help individuals value and believe in themselves.

- Support is given to adopt healthy behaviours in relation to diet and exercise (DH 2002).

- Seminars are given to provide health education on sexual health and communicable diseases, for example, advice on sexually transmitted diseases. In some prisons peer education groups have been established by prisoners, and these groups have organized days to raise awareness of diseases such as HIV and AIDS (DH 2002).

Activity

- Compare the information provided above from the Social Exclusion Unit (2002) with case scenario 4: David.

- Does this information help your understanding of why David, by the age of 27, has served a number of prison terms?

Application to practice

Case scenario 4: David

David could be empowered to make the decision to change his health-related behaviour through the following types of health promotion activities:

- Health education on the benefits of not smoking and not abusing drugs could be provided.

- Education alone would not mean that David would choose to change his lifestyle, and therefore the behavioural approach discussed earlier in this chapter would also be useful.

- David could be encouraged to engage in physical exercise.

- The mental health nurse has organized for David to engage in meaningful occupation by working in the prison kitchen. This would help develop his self-esteem, confidence and skills that might be useful in future employment.

> • David has also been offered a place in a reading class, which would develop personal skills, and facilitate understanding of the benefits of not abusing drugs or smoking. This could also impact on his feelings of self-worth.

Hospitals and enablement centres (rehabilitation units)

Hospitals and enablement centres have a role in promoting the health of the population. Admissions to hospital and enablement centres are due to numerous reasons such as following a heart attack, stroke or treatment for cancer or diabetes or for mental health reasons. Health promotion work needs to be included alongside medical intervention and rehabilitation. A needs assessment must be included; for example, an assessment of health-related behaviours such as unhealthy diet, smoking, drug or alcohol abuse and lack of exercise; evidence suggests that these behaviours can lead to the reasons for admission given above (Sanderson et al. 2009; Wainwright et al. 2007). Making the decision to change health-related behaviour and successfully achieving this change takes time, therefore on discharge it is essential that support is given to facilitate change and maintenance of change.

The provision of information on local support services should therefore be a requirement. If health promotion is provided at the secondary level (Chapter 2) then support services provide a key role in preventing readmission rates (Hubley and Copeman 2008; Naidoo and Wills 2009).

Hospitals and enablement centres can work with primary health care practices, communities and schools in promoting health and well-being and involving patients in decisions related to their care can lead to improved patient outcomes (Coulter 2002, cited in Naidoo and Wills 2009).

Application to practice

Case scenario 3: Richard

Richard could be empowered to make the decision to change his health-related behaviour through the following types of health promotion activities:

- health education on the benefits of regular cholesterol checks and the benefits of not smoking and moderate drinking;
- stress management;
- development of coping strategies;
- diet management, including development of cooking skills;
- job searching and interview skills in case he wants to change direction.

Health promotion initiatives have incorporated the proposal for smoke-free hospital environments in a number of countries. Following the ninth international conference on health promoting hospitals held in 2001 (Groene and Barbero 2005) a working group was established to identify core standards for hospitals and rehabilitation services. In all, five standards were identified:

1   Hospital policy on including health promotion should be implemented as part of quality management programmes.

2   Following needs assessment, health promotion activities should be included to promote health and well-being.

3   Health promotion initiatives should be included as part of integrated care pathways that would empower individuals to make the decision to change their health-related behaviour.

4   Health promotion is equally important to patients and employees and therefore organizations must ensure the workplace is a healthy place to work.

5   There should be collaboration with relevant providers.

Community

There is some tension when considering health promotion within communities. Policies identified by the government may conflict with the priorities of communities, who may base health promotion on the social model and not the medical model. The standards above state the importance of collaboration; however, this is not necessarily easy to establish due to the number of organizations within a community (Hubley and Copeman 2008).

Having said this, a number of community health promotion initiatives have been organized. Here are three examples:

1   The NHS Forth Valley Health Promotion Department awards grants that enable local communities to develop health promotion activities, for example, to build raised beds for service users to grow vegetables and then cook healthy meals under supervision. They also run monthly drop-in cookery groups for service users to develop skills (NHS Forth Valley 2011).

2   Derbyshire County Council has run a number of initiatives within community settings to promote sexual health through peer support. For example, small groups of young people are provided with information on communicable diseases such as chlamydia and HIV in order to support their peers. Initiatives have been organized in local pubs or clubs where individuals may feel more comfortable asking questions (Derbyshire County Council 2009).

3   Falkirk City Council (2011) has arranged the Big Fit Walk since 2003, in which the local community is encouraged to take part in walking events. One of the key aims of these events is to raise awareness of the benefits that exercise has on individual health. A step-by-step guide is provided by the council to help community groups organize walks and walking 'meetings' can be organized where teams are divided up to discuss particular issues.

Activity

Identify another example of a community initiative taking place near where you work.

- What is the aim of this initiative?

- Who is involved?

- How has this initiative been organized?

- Are there any resource implications?

Application to practice

Case scenario 2: Hamed

This scenario illustrates how Hamed's wife Halima identified some health-related priorities. First of all she noticed that Hamed had put on weight and was continually thirsty. She then noticed a poster in the local surgery which supported her concerns that Hamed may have diabetes. Halima then sought support from the practice nurse who made an appointment for Hamed to go and see her. Part of the support offered was a referral to a community support group for newly diagnosed diabetics.

Chapter summary

In this chapter, we have illustrated the diverse nature of health promotion activities and the many places in which it takes place, for example, schools, prisons, enablement centres, communities and hospitals. Considering the contexts and ideas will help you to understand a number of aspects for exploration. Therefore, when planning health promotion work with an individual or group of individuals, you will need to think about the situation and then which approach(es) – i.e. educational, behavioural, medical, societal or empowerment – could be used. You will also need to think about which level of health promotion is appropriate – primary, secondary or tertiary.

Implications for practice

- Health promotion is much wider than simply providing health education through providing information, and therefore you need to recognize the scope of health promotion in order to understand its relevance to your role.

- Health promotion can take place within schools, hospitals and enablement centres, communities and prisons, so you need to acknowledge the varied contexts where health promotion work is carried out because of its diverse nature, and you will need to work with a variety of professionals as well as clients.

- It is also important for you to use theory to underpin your practice, and to understand how approaches and levels of health promotion will impact on choices of health promotion work in practice.

Key points

- Health promotion includes a wide variety of activities other than just health education.

- There are a variety of approaches to health promotion and selection of approach depends on the situation.

- Health promotion takes place in a wide variety of settings.

End of chapter questions

1 How does an understanding of the definitions of health promotion help you to develop your practice?

2 How can the health promotion activities be influenced by the approach(es) and levels?

3 How can government directives, e.g. healthy eating in schools, help you in your role as a health promoter?

References

Derbyshire City Council (2009) *Sexual Health Promotion Service Peer Education Initiative.* http://www.idea.gov.uk/idk/core/page.do?pageId=14342334 (accessed 20 September 2011).

Department for Education (2011) *Healthy Schools Tool Kit.* http://www.education.gov.uk/schools/pupilsupport/pastoralcare/a0075278/healthy-schools (accessed 5 September 2011).

DH (Department of Health) (2009) *Change4Life:* www.dh.gov.uk/en/AdvanceSearchResult/index.htm?searchTerms=DoH+change4life (accessed 20 September 2011).

DH (Department of Health) (2002) *Health Promoting Prisons: A Shared Approach.* London: HMSO.

Falkirk City Council (2011) *Big Fit Walk.* http://www.falkirk.gov.uk/services/trust/fitness/circuit_health_club/step_forth/big_fit_walk/big_fit_walk.aspx (accessed 20 September 2011).

Gatherer, A., Moller, L. and Hayton, P. (2005) The World Health Organisation European Health in Prisons project after 10 years: persistent barriers and achievements. *American Journal of Public Health,* 95 (10): 1696–700.

Groene, O. and Barbero, G. (eds) (2005) *Health Promotion in Hospitals: Evidence and Quality Management.* Copenhagen: World Health Organisation.

Hubley, J. and Copeman, J. (2008) *Practical Health Promotion.* Cambridge: Polity.

Lee, A., Cheng F., Yuen, H. et al. (2007) Achieving good standards in health promoting schools: preliminary analysis one year after the implementation of the Hong Kong Healthy Schools Award scheme. *Public Health,* 121: 752–60.

Naidoo, J. and Wills, J. (2000) *Health Promotion: Foundations for Practice.* London: Baillière Tindall.

Naidoo, J. and Wills, J. (2009) *Public Health and Health Promotion Practice: Foundations for Health Promotion.* London: Bailliere Tindall Elsevier.

NHS Forth Valley (2011) *Bringing Health Care Closer to your Home.* http://www.nhsforthvalley.com/home/Services/healthpromotion/hp_intro.html (accessed 21 September 2011).

Peixoto, R. (2010) Associations between health promoting schools' policies and indicators of oral health in Brazil. *Health Promotion International,* 18 (3): 209–18.

Rana, L. and Alvaro, R. (2010) Applying a health promoting schools approach to nutrition interventions in schools: key factors to success. *Health Promotion Journal of Australia,* 21(2): 106–13.

Sanderson, S.C., Waller, J., Jarvis, M., Humphries, S.E. and Wardle, J. (2009) Awareness of lifestyle risk factors for cancer and heart disease among adults in the UK. *Patient Education and Counseling,* 74: 221–7.

Scriven, A. (2010) *Promoting Health: A Practical Guide.* London: Baillière Tindall Elsevier.

Seedhouse, D. (2001) *Health: Foundations for Achievement,* 2nd edn. Chichester: John Wiley.

Social Exclusion Unit (2002) *Report: Reducing Re-offending by Ex Prisoners.* London: Social Exclusion Unit.

Wainwright, N., Surtees, P., Welch, A. et al. (2007) Healthy lifestyle choices: could sense of coherence aid health promotion? *Journal of Epidemiology and Community Health,* 61(10): 871–6.

WHO (World Health Organisation) (1986) *The Ottawa Charter*. http://www.who.int/hpr/
NPH/docs/ottawa_charter_hp.pdf (accessed 9 March 2012).

Useful resources

'Brief interventions and referral for smoking cessation' (NICE public health guidance 1)
'Behaviour change' (NICE public health guidance 6)
'School-based interventions on alcohol' (NICE public health guidance 7)
'Personal, social and health education focusing on sex and relationships and alcohol guid-
    ance (NICE public health guidance).
https://www.Nice.org.uk/guidance23
http://www.education.gov.uk/schools/pupilsupport/pastoralcare/a0075278/healthy-schools
http://www.nhs.uk/change4llfe/Pages/partner-tools.aspx
http://www.nhsforthvalley.com/home/Services/healthpromotion/hp_intro.html
http://www.idea.gov.uk/idk/core/page.do?pageId=14342334
http://www.falkirk.gov.uk/services/trust/fitness/circuit_health_club/step_forth/big_fit_walk/
    bigfit_walk.aspx

Part 2

Empowering individuals and communities

3

Health Promotion Models and Application to Practice

Mary Gottwald and Jane Goodman-Brown

Chapter contents

Introduction

The previous chapter identified a number of complexities to consider. Approaches to health promotion can guide practice, however information alone (education approach) does not lead to behavioural change and, as highlighted by Naidoo and Wills (2009), it can be difficult to prove that there is a link between the intervention and any subsequent change (behavioural approach). This chapter will consider models of behaviour change; these can also be useful to us when planning health promotion programmes, as they are a way of linking theory and practice, and assist us to plan and implement health promotion interventions.

Health promotion, as already discussed, can involve individuals making decisions to change their health behaviour and adopt healthy behaviours. However, it is suggested that information on its own does not necessarily lead to change

(Bundy 2004). Understanding why information alone does not always lead to change has led to the development of a variety of models.

This chapter will consider three models of behavioural change, namely the Stages of Change Model, Health Action Model and Health Belief Model. The Stages of Change Model will be applied to David (case scenario 4). The Health Action Model will be applied to Emily (case scenario 1) and the Health Belief Model will be applied to Hamed (case scenario 2). We will also discuss how motivational interviewing links to the Stages of Change Model, and will apply this to Richard (case scenario 3). Examples of health promotion activities will be suggested; however, these will be explored and discussed in more depth in the next two chapters.

Learning objectives

By the end of this chapter the reader will be better able to:

- Identify and apply behavioural change models to practice

- Compare and contrast models

- Understand how motivational interviewing can facilitate change

- Understand how motivational interviewing links to models of practice

Stages of Change Model (Transtheoretical Model)

Although Prochaska and DiClemente (1982) initially described this model as a linear model, it is more widely known as a circular model (Figure 3.1). The advantage of the circular model is that it acknowledges that it is not easy to immediately change health-related behaviour, for example having multiple partners without using condoms; smoking; abusing drugs; or eating an unhealthy diet. Reasons for this could be due to addictions or external social and environmental influences, such as unemployment, poor accommodation or the impact of tsunamis or earthquakes that we discussed in Chapter 1.

Prochaska and Di Clemente (1982) suggest that individuals go through a number of stages before successfully changing their health-related behaviour, and that time frames within each stage will vary. There are five stages that individuals will go through in order to successfully change their health-related behaviour,

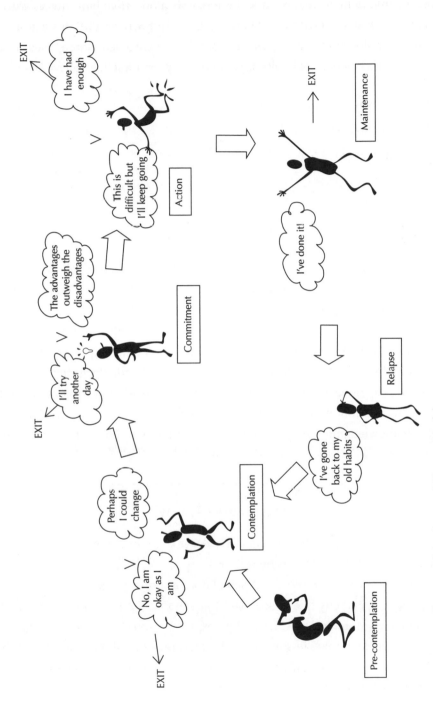

Figure 3.1 Application of the Stages of Change Model
Source: adapted from Prochaska and DiClemente (1984)

however some individuals, in particular those with addictive behaviours, will go through a sixth stage. Ewles and Simnett (2003) and Scriven (2010) suggest that those trying to stop smoking may well go round the cycle at least three times before succeeding. This theory could also be applied to other addictive behaviours:

1 pre-contemplation
2 contemplation
3 commitment
4 action
5 maintenance
6 relapse

Different terminology is used for the third stage; Anderson et al. (1999) and Prochaska et al. (1992) use 'preparation' and Scriven (2010) uses 'commitment'. In this book we are going to use 'commitment'.

It is essential that we recognize and respect an individual's autonomy. Even though an individual may understand the benefits of not smoking, of losing weight, of engaging in 'safe' sexual activities, they may also make the decision to continue their unhealthy behaviour(s). If an individual does decide not to continue with their health promotion programme, we must still show support; so we could do this by acknowledging their decision and giving them a contact number should they wish to have another go at a later stage.

Case scenario 4: David

Before we can apply this model to David, it is important to consider the reasons that have led to his behaviour.

David's school life was not straightforward and he was labelled as having a hyperactivity disorder whilst at school. He left school without gaining any qualifications. These are possible reasons that have led to his unemployment, homelessness and ultimately prison. Although his mother does visit him when in prison, when she can afford to, there would appear to be limited family support.

Application to practice

Case scenario 4: David

Pre-contemplation

Individuals in this stage are not intending to change *or* are not aware of the importance of changing. David is not in this stage because he has signed up for a smoking cessation group. If he was in this stage it would be essential not to focus on him personally and so the aim of health promotion would be to 'raise awareness'.

This could be achieved by

> **Key point**
>
> Assessing whether the individual is ready to change

- focusing on the general benefits of not smoking and not abusing drugs, in other words the focus is not on David per se;

- discussing the disadvantages of smoking/abusing drugs;

- providing a leaflet and/or a contact number. It is important to check the level of language used in the leaflets as David has a learning difficulty;

- offering unconditional support.

Contemplation

In this stage, individuals are aware that they have a problem and therefore are thinking about changing. Again we can say that David is not in this stage because he has joined a smoking cessation group. If he were in this stage health promotion activities could include:

> **Key point**
>
> Identifying activities that will facilitate the individual to move to the next stage

- the health promoter discussing the advantages and disadvantages in relation to David; this would facilitate problem solving and decision making. This discussion could link to his recent cough;

- it is important to continue to focus on the benefits of not smoking/ abusing drugs;

- problem solving: a decision balance matrix table could be used to help David identify the advantages and disadvantages of his health-related behaviours and this could help him to prioritize which aspects of his behaviour he would like to change first of all. (An example of this tool will be included in the discussion on motivational interviewing later in this chapter.)

- acknowledgement that changing behaviour is not easy, and providing opportunities for David to voice his concerns about stopping smoking;

- offer of future support/follow-up appointment.

Commitment (preparation)

We can say that David is in this stage because he is 'beginning to stop smoking'. He is also taking part in a needle exchange clinic. It is impor-

Key point

David identifies his goals

tant in this stage that David identifies some goals for himself and for him to set a 'stop smoking date'. We can work alongside David to ensure that his goals are achievable and the time frame realistic. So far he has been faced with numerous challenges in his life and therefore may have low self-esteem, and lack assertiveness and confidence.

Individuals who lack assertiveness, confidence and have low self-esteem may well not move to the next stage. In order to facilitate this move, health promotion activities could include:

- discussions and acknowledgement of his concerns;

- development of these life skills; for example, role play could help David to become more assertive to say 'no' to a cigarette or drugs. Being able to say 'no' will improve his self-esteem and confidence;

- identification of any potential barriers such as boredom. If David has no job and is homeless, this could well lead to boredom and lack of motivation;

- offering counselling;

- identifying strategies that would not encourage further bullying (due to his learning difficulty he may be teased or bullied);

- provision of nicotine replacement therapy (NRT), for example, NRT patches, chewing gum or nicotine inhaler;

- the prison doctor prescribing Zyban (medication that facilitates giving up smoking). However, like other medications this could cause side effects such as insomnia;

- motivational interviewing (see the section below that discusses this).

Action

When David reaches this stage he will have stopped smoking and may well have agreed to take up his place on the detox programme. Too many changes may be difficult and therefore it is essential that we respect his autonomy in that he may well be continuing to take part in the needle exchange programme as opposed to the detox programme.

Health promotion activities could include:

> **Key point**
>
> David to prioritize the changes he wishes to make

- helping David to identify strategies that work for him, for example, saving the money that he would have spent on cigarettes. He could treat himself at a later date. Staff need to acknowledge success because this will increase his self-esteem and confidence;

- relaxation techniques to help reduce stress, e.g. breathing exercises or yoga;

- stress management techniques can be effective and can help the decision to avoid smoking or abusing drugs, e.g. listening to music, exercise;

- improving his reading could improve his confidence and self-esteem;

- developing his confidence further by setting more achievable goals;

- encouraging different hobbies, for example, taking up more exercise, learning to cook;

- David may well be putting on weight at this point, because giving up smoking can lead to weight gain as smoking is an appetite suppressant. He now works in the prison kitchen and therefore staff could help him to understand the importance of a balanced diet;

- developing his cookery skills could help David once he is released from prison;

- keeping a diary would encourage David to monitor his behaviour and staff could then discuss with him the triggers that cause him to smoke.

Maintenance

Key point

Changing health behaviours takes time and David may be facing different challenges at this point

By the time David reaches this stage he may well have been released from prison and therefore this could be a really challenging stage. Although he will have stopped smoking for some time now, it is essential that support continues on his release and it is clear from the scenario that he has already been promised this support.

Health promotion activities could include:

- helping David identify strategies that have helped him so far;

- stress management, relaxation techniques and, if needed, anger management. He may well get himself into difficult social situations. such as arguments, which could lead him to start smoking again;

- offering him the opportunity to join a community support group for those who have given up smoking (former addicts) or are still aiming to do so;

- providing the number of a support hot line;

- agreeing a follow-up appointment; this could be face to face or a telephone conversation. It is important for David to know that there is still support available if he wants it.

Relapse

Research evidence acknowledges that David may not maintain the changes that he has made while in prison and therefore may revert back to the Contemplation stage of the Stages of Change Model (Ewles and Simnett 2003).

Key point

Relapse is a normal part of change

Health promotion activities need to:

- make sure that David does not feel that he has failed. He may feel guilty and ashamed so it is important that he understands that it is normal to go through this cycle more than once. He also needs to know that support is unconditional and will continue;

- discuss what led to him to start smoking again;

- identify strategies that have worked so far;

- encourage David to return to the contemplation stage or action stage. He may feel that he does not need to go 'back to the beginning'.

Table 3.1 outlines the advantages and disadvantages of the Stages of Change Model.

Activity

Think of someone you work with or someone you know.

- Is this a useful model to guide your practice with this individual?

- What health promotion activities could you incorporate into each stage that would facilitate this person moving on to the next stage?

Table 3.1   Critique of the Stages of Change Model

Advantages	Disadvantages
A simple model	Does not give practitioners ideas on HOW to facilitate individuals moving from one stage to the next, i.e. does not suggest any specific health promotion activities
Helps us to identify when individuals are ready to make the decision to change	
Acknowledges that individuals go through a number of stages before succeeding	
There are no specified time frames for each stage	The boundaries between stages may not be clear
Helps us to recognize that time frames for each individual will vary	Difficult to assess when someone is 'ready' to change
Evidence to support that this is a popular and successful resource and easy to apply in practice	No specified time frames for each stage and therefore this lack of structure may not be easy for some individuals
Evidence to support the use of this model with addictive behaviours	
Can be applied in any context	
Acknowledges that individuals may relapse and revert back to their unhealthy behaviours	

Source: West (2005); Hubley and Copeman (2008); Naidoo and Wills (2009)

Stop and think

- Can you think of any other advantages of this model?
- Can you identify any other disadvantages of this model?
- Do you think this model supports David to lead a healthier lifestyle?
- If so, what has led you to make this decision?
- Are there any barriers that would lead David to continuing with smoking, drug and alcohol abuse?

Motivational interviewing

Motivational interviewing is a specialized technique originating from the addictions field (Miller and Rollnick 2002). It is a technique to explore ambivalence to change with clients so that they can make an informed decision, being aware of the benefits of change and the difficulties of changing rather than being persuaded by professionals to do something they may not want to do. It is often used alongside the Stages of Change Model to establish whether someone is ready to change.

Motivational interviewing is different to the traditional approach to behaviour change. In the traditional approach professionals give information, advise clients and help them to develop their skills so they can change their behaviour in order to solve a health problem. Focusing on advice, information and skills implies that health itself is a motivator for people to change but this may not be the case (Hillsdon 2006): in fact it often leads to resistance to change as people feel the need to defend their current behaviour. For example, in smoking cessation giving advice on the benefits of quitting to someone who is not interested in stopping smoking might lead them to tell you about their great uncle who smoked 40 cigarettes a day and lived to be 104. They are trying to defend their position as they are not ready to change their behaviour.

Motivational interviewing takes a different approach and tries to help clients to explore why they are not ready to change and how this links to their views on life. By doing this the technique overcomes ambivalence and clients can then be given advice and support to help them change. It recognizes that in order to change our behaviour we have to change our feelings and beliefs linked to that behaviour.

Key points

Motivational interviewing explores ambivalence to change

Advice, information and skills development do not necessarily lead to change

Stop and think

Reflect on your practice. Can you remember an occasion when you have tried to help someone change and have met with resistance?

Principles involved in motivational interviewing

There are five recognized principles of motivational interviewing which are used to assess and create motivation in individuals (Miller and Rollnick 2002). We will use a very brief case scenario to illustrate these principles and will then apply the process to Richard.

Jane

Jane is a 40-year-old woman who is 3 stone overweight and takes a size 18 dress. She loves to eat cakes and biscuits and has frequent snacks. She has tried numerous diets but is unable to comply with them so doesn't lose weight. She has a goal of being able to fit into a size 12 dress for her wedding in six months' time.

Principle 1: express empathy

Basically this means listening reflectively to what someone has to say about their behaviour and accepting that this is the way it is for them; it is a way of trying to understand and accept their situation. For example, to express empathy with Jane you would listen to how she describes her diet including the frequent snacks. You might say to her 'I can hear how much you enjoy your food and how difficult it is for you to change'. The idea is to convey interest and acceptance of the person and their situation. It is not helpful to be judgemental. It is more effective if you listen and try to understand how it is for Jane without trying to get her to change.

Principle 2: avoid arguments

Although motivational interviewing involves challenge and confrontation about behaviour it does not include arguments between the practitioner and client. So if Jane believes she can't change, you should not argue with her as she probably believes this is true. Instead you should help her to see that change is possible through discussion and examples.

Principle 3: develop a discrepancy

This is how people are motivated to change, by identifying that there is discrepancy between what they are doing and what they would like to achieve. The client, in this case Jane, should be encouraged to identify their own goal. For Jane it is wearing her dream dress. The discrepancy is identifying the gap between where they are now and where they want to be. Once the client accepts that there is a discrepancy they can start to change. Identifying this evolves as part of a therapeutic conversation and developing a relationship. This links to communication skills in Chapter 5, which will help with this.

Principle 4: roll with resistance

Often when talking to a client about change they are resistant to it. In motivational interviewing it is important not to try to persuade them to change but to accept their resistance. It is important not to confront resistance but to accept it. If at the end of the discussion, Jane makes the decision that she does not want to lose weight her autonomy must be respected.

Principle 5: supporting self-efficacy

This means that clients need to believe in themselves and their ability to change. The more self-belief an individual has the more likely they are to be able to change (Bandura 2004). This is achieved by encouraging clients to be positive about what they want to achieve. Sometimes changing thinking from 'I can't do it' to 'I can' will help to change actions. The role of the health promoter is to help identify the positive statements and to help the client to believe they can change (Bundy 2004). It can also be helpful to identify others who have been successful and to offer support. For Jane this might include discussing her experiences of weight loss and identifying positives as well as giving examples of others who have been successful in losing weight and offering her support to try and achieve her goal.

> **Key points**
>
> Motivational interviewing helps to identify Jane's readiness to change
>
> This is the equivalent of contemplation in the Stages of Change Model

Motivational interviewing: underlying ideas

Miller and Rollnick (2002) suggest that there are three fundamental ideas under-lying any consultation using motivational interviewing:

- There should be a spirit of collaboration between the practitioner and client.

- Motivation for change should come from the client.

- The client's autonomy should be respected.

From reading the discussion above you can see how this is applied in using moti-vational interviewing with Jane.

Ideas and principles are all very well but as busy health promoters practical steps are also useful. Miller and Rollnick (2002) describe eight steps which enable motivational interviewing to be effective. They are:

1   establishing rapport

2   setting the agenda

3   assessing readiness to change

4   sharpening the focus

5   identifying ambivalence

6   eliciting self-motivation statements

7   handling resistance

8   shifting the focus

Application to practice

Case scenario 3: Richard

Step 1: Establishing a rapport

To help Richard explore his health behaviours it is important to set aside time and to agree a venue where he feels comfortable. This may not be before his discharge home as it might be better in the community. There should be a clear time scale for the session and time should be spent getting to know each other and agreeing ground rules.

Key points

Set aside time
Plan a time scale for the session

Step 2: Setting the agenda

It should be Richard who decides which issues he wants to address in order to improve his health. He might want to stop smoking or take more exercise but he should set his own goals and these should be reviewed regularly. You can help him make decisions by using open-ended questions such as 'how do you feel about your smoking'?

Step 3: Assessing readiness to change

There are a variety of techniques for this, for example, a decisional balance or a rating scale (see Table 3.2). Using a rating scale you can ask Richard to rate his readiness to stop smoking on a scale of 1–10. If he says 5 it is important to probe why it is a 5 rather than a 6. This helps to show discrepancy in his view and his readiness and willingness to change (contemplation/commitment in the Stages of Change Model). Doing this helps to develop collaboration and to respect his autonomy as motivational interviewing should be a transparent process.

Step 4: Sharpening the focus

Having identified what Richard wants to change it is then essential to be precise. If Richard wants to stop smoking then this should be the focus with Richard identifying achievable goals such as:
'By the end of (date) I will have reduced my daily cigarette consumption to 10 a day'.
Behaviour is the result of habits and so it helps to break the habits down into manageable parts and change a bit at a time. It might be that Richard

Key points

Allow time to get to know each other
Allow Richard to decide the issues
Allow Richard to identify his goals
Use open-ended questions

usually smokes his first cigarette when he has his first coffee; he could change this habit and maybe stop having a cigarette. You can help him with this by affirming his choice, for example, if he says he is concerned that his smoking might be damaging his health you can agree with this by saying 'you are right to be concerned smoking can damage your health'. By using this technique you are not judging him you are helping to build a relationship with him.

Step 5: Identifying ambivalence

Richard could be encouraged to consider how he feels in relation to change by identifying what he is concerned about in relation to change and exploring ideas about why he should change but also why he might not want to change.

Step 6: Eliciting self-motivating statements

Richard could be encouraged to be positive and to identify his successes. So if he changes his early morning coffee and doesn't have a cigarette this is a success and should be acknowledged rather than him thinking 'I have only given up one cigarette'. You can help him to make positive statements about what he is doing and then explore these with him. For example he might say 'if only I could stop my lunchtime cigarettes': he could reframe this into a positive 'I would like to stop my lunchtime cigarettes'. Reframing is an important part of motivational interviewing. Helping individuals to see the progress they have made by making sure you feed back their success to them is also helpful.

Step 7: Handling resistance

Because we behave in a certain way for a reason, there is often resistance to change, as discussed above in relation to Jane. This, like ambivalence, is normal. However as a promoter we need to be able to address this. If Richard misses appointments it is important to find out why and what the problem is rather than trying to persuade him to continue. This should be addressed through reflection. This will help him to develop his coping skills and enable him to overcome obstacles.

Step 8: Shifting the focus

This can be another way of handling resistance. Sometimes it is about identifying barriers and trying to help the client to overcome them. If Richard says he misses appointments because it is difficult to find time to attend, it is important to discuss why this is a barrier to him changing his behaviour through open questions and reflection. However, it is important not to confront him or to try to persuade him to change.

(Adapted from Miller and Rollnick 2002; Registered Nurses Association of Ontario 2007)

Motivational interviewing helps individuals understand why they behave in a particular way and it helps them to identify whether they want to change and if so how. Your role in this is to support them in their decisions, not to tell them what to do.

Table 3.2   Decisional balance matrix – application to drinking less

Changing behaviour – drinking less	*Remaining the same*
Benefits	**Benefits**
Feel better	Remain relaxed
Have more energy	
Costs	**Costs**
Less relaxed	Long-term effects on health
Need another way of coping with stress	

Activity

Skills for motivational interviewing

Motivational interviewing uses a range of skills, many of which health professionals already have:

- reflection

- empathy

- reframing

- open-ended questions

- affirmation

- self-motivational statements

- personal feedback

Look back at the discussion in relation to Richard and see if you can find examples of these skills.

Brief interventions

Motivational interviewing was designed to be part of a therapeutic relationship and takes time to achieve change. Each encounter is presumed to be about an hour. For many health promoters, whatever their role, this is unrealistic. Motivational interviewing has been adapted into brief interventions to take account of this, which might be more practical in some situations.

NICE (2006) public health guidance illustrates a brief intervention for smoking cessation. It begins by suggesting that health professionals ask clients or patients if they smoke every time they have contact, e.g. at an appointment about something else, or if they have a chance meeting and then follow this up with brief succinct advice.

If they answer yes to the question 'do you smoke?', the first stage is to ask if they want to stop.

- If they reply 'yes' to this explain the services available to them.

- If they say 'no' accept their decision but offer support if they want to stop in the future. This offer should be renewed annually.

- If they want to stop you can refer them to

  - intensive support

  - nicotine replacement therapy

  - advice on how to stop and details of the help line.

Whichever option they choose should be followed up and their decision supported.

Like many brief interventions, this intervention focuses on being an opportunistic encounter where the purpose is to initiate thinking about change in behaviour. It tends to be more directed than motivational interviewing with less emphasis on choice and personal responsibility (Hillsdon 2006).

Activity

- Can you think of an example of using a brief intervention approach to behaviour change?

- Was it successful?

- Why was it successful/why wasn't it successful?

One of the criticisms of brief interventions is that they are only loosely based on motivational interviewing and as such do not have such an established evidence base as pure motivational interviewing.

Health Belief Model

This is a social cognition model which focuses on understanding an individual's perceptions of reality rather than how they respond to their situation (Abraham et al. 2008). Therefore it considers why people make the decision to change and what sustains this decision; it is based on perceptions as opposed to reactions to events. It was one of the first social cognition theories developed by American social psychologists and it was initially developed to try and help explain why individuals did not attend for free screening tests (Becker 1974; Hochbaum 1958, cited in Green and Tones 2010). Its focus is to help people to understand and alter their own beliefs and is one of the most commonly used health promotion models (Green and Tones 2010).

Key point

This model focuses on individual perceptions

This model suggests that individuals base their health-related behaviours and decisions on six major beliefs, which are listed below and discussed.

- **Perceived susceptibility** – the belief that they are susceptible to the disease or event.

- **Perceived seriousness** – the belief that the disease or event is serious.

- **Perceived benefits** – the belief that taking action will reduce their susceptibility to and the severity of the disease or event.

- **Perceived barriers** – the belief that the benefits of the change outweigh the costs.

- **Cues to action** – prompts that change the health behaviour. An example of this might be if a peer who you thought was not susceptible to heart disease was diagnosed with the disease. This may cause you to assess your own risks and change your behaviour. Or exposure to a 'cue to action', such as health advice from a health professional as demonstrated in Hamed's situation below.

- **Health motivation** – the value that is placed on health and ability to influence this, for example, whether or not someone feels that they are able to affect their health (Abraham et al. 2008).

Later versions of the model known as the 'extended health belief model' (Pender et al. 2011) include self-efficacy which is confidence in one's own ability to take health action (Rimmer and Glanz 2005). This is the version that is being discussed in this chapter. Understanding how the different elements of the model work together is illustrated in Figure 3.2. The model highlights that the likelihood of an individual taking action depends on all of the factors being addressed. If a change is to be implemented successfully, the individual needs to balance whether or not they think

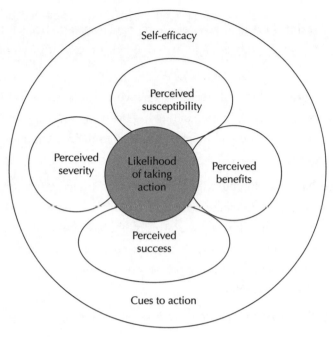

Figure 3.2 Health Belief Model
Source: Adapted from Goodman-Brown and Gottwald (2008)

they are likely to be harmed or are susceptible to harm as a result of their behaviour, then need to consider what the individual benefits of change are and compare these with any individual costs. For example if they are considering giving up smoking, they should balance the health benefits of stopping with the costs of giving up smoking such as increased stress. Furthermore the decision to change will be influenced by their self-belief and whether or not they think they will be successful. The model suggests that external cues can also influence the decision to change.

Application to practice

Case scenario 2: Hamed

Perceived susceptibility Hamed needs to believe that he is susceptible to diabetes in order to help him change his behaviour. He might well believe he is susceptible as his father had diabetes and Hamed has high blood sugar.

Perceived seriousness Hamed needs to recognize that diabetes is likely to affect his health; he has already experienced some of the symptoms of diabetes.

Perceived benefits Hamed needs to believe that a change in diet will control his symptoms. A change in diet has been suggested. Attending the support group where he will meet others in a similar situation might help him to change his behaviour.

Perceived barriers Hamed enjoys his food and his wife is a traditional cook. To help control his diabetes it is important that Hamed eats healthily and Halima cooks in a healthy way. This might have cultural implications for the family and the adjustments might be difficult. Therefore involving Halima from the beginning is important so that she can be supported and in turn can support Hamed

Cues to action Hamed has experienced some of the signs and symptoms of diabetes. He has been feeling generally unwell, and Halima has been his main cue to action, by making him an appointment with the practice nurse to find out what is wrong.

Self-efficacy From the scenario it is clear that Halima is proactive and values Hamed's health. It is unclear how confident Hamed is about change, but he did attend the appointment with the nurse which is positive. However, he has shown that he can be proactive in his business life and so he might be able to transfer these skills to his health.

Health promotion activities

Key point

Health beliefs will affect health behaviours

From applying the model to Hamed's situation it would seem that he believes change is possible. This can help a health promoter to suggest possible activities such as:

- a support group
- cookery demonstrations
- increasing the family's knowledge of diabetes.

It also highlights the areas that require extra work such as increasing Hamed's **self-efficacy**, possibly by helping him to become more confident through training in how to be more assertive and through giving information about where to get help.

Explanation of how the Health Belief Model works

Green and Tones (2010) suggest that the model is based on decision making being influenced by the expectation that following a particular course of action will lead to a desirable result. Therefore if the beliefs are fulfilled the model predicts that a changed health behaviour will be adopted by an individual, so according to this model Hamed is likely to try to change his behaviour. The model can help in planning effective behaviour change strategies for individuals and communities.

However Naidoo and Wills (2009) comment that people's perception of their own risk from a disease is influenced by their personal experience, their ability to control the situation and a fear that a disease is a killer. They go on to suggest that people are often overly optimistic about their invulnerability to disease and so are unrealistic, which affects the likelihood of them changing their behaviour.

Activity

- Think of a patient/client you have worked with.

- How would the Health Belief Model help you to understand the likelihood of them changing their health behaviour?

Table 3.3 outlines the advantages and disadvantages of the Health Belief Model.

Even though it has its disadvantages (see Table 3.3), the Health Belief Model can be a useful model as indicated above in the scenario. It can help with planning individual interventions through highlighting areas for consideration (Green and Tones 2010; Naidoo and Wills 2009). Therefore it is a practical model to use when working with individuals.

Table 3.3   Advantages and disadvantages of using the Health Belief Model

Advantages	*Disadvantages*
It predicts whether an individual might take preventative action, e.g. attend for screening.	It assumes health decisions are made rationally.
It helps to predict whether someone might change their behaviour.	It takes a bio-medical view of health.
It illustrates the importance of individual beliefs and it explores how change in beliefs might lead to a change in behaviour.	The evidence that the model is effective in relation to health behaviours such as alcohol misuse or smoking is limited.
It helps an individual to explore the costs and benefits of any action.	It does not acknowledge the wider determinants of heath.
It illustrates the complex nature of decision making and the range of factors that affect change.	It does not recognize the role of family, social life, cultural environment and political factors.
It is perceived barriers followed by susceptibility that are the two most important dimensions in predicting change.	It does not recognize that not all cues to action have the same weighting, for example a poster will not have the same impact as a relative becoming unwell.

Source: Green and Tones (2010); Naidoo and Wills (2009); Pender et al. (2010)

Health Action Model

This model (see Figure 3.3) is also not a new model and was introduced by Tones in the 1970s. Initially it appears to be more complex than the Stages of Change Model or Health Belief Model; however, it is useful in that it guides our thinking and helps us to analyse a number of different aspects that could influence an individual's intentions to change.

Explanation of the Health Action Model

There are two key aspects that we need first to consider:

1   Behavioural intention: the individual's intention to change. For example an individual may have the intention to stop smoking but the outcome may depend on a number of factors such as a lack of assertiveness skills or smoking to relieve stress.

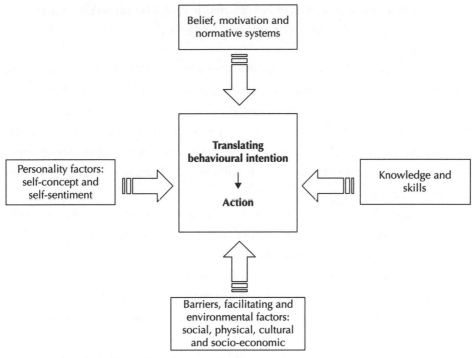

Figure 3.3 Health Action Model
Source: Adapted from Goodman-Brown and Gottwald (2008) and Tones and Tilford (2001)

2 Translating intention into action: the individual changes their health-related behaviour, gives up smoking and sustains the change.

There are also three systems that we need to consider. These systems can influence whether an individual is likely to translate their intention into action:

1 Belief system: this relates to how the individual receives information, for example, does the individual understand the importance of stopping smoking from a factual perspective? Providing health education through leaflets will influence their belief systems.

2 Motivation system: this concerns the individual's value system and attitudes and feelings about an issue, for example, does Emily's mother value weight loss and will it make her and Emily happier?

3 Normative system: norms are accepted rules of behaviour within a group or society and have cognitive and affective elements. If everyone in the

family smokes or is overweight then it could be more difficult to stop because this would not be considered the norm.

The belief system and motivation system are interconnected because information received and understood may create new beliefs. So if an individual receives information that provides evidence that stopping smoking increases life chances then they may value this for themselves. If Emily's mother is provided with information that links weight loss to happiness then she may value this change. However, if they do not believe that it will make a difference to their lives then they may block any new information.

The Health Action Model goes on to acknowledge that personality (i.e. self-concept and self-sentiment) could influence translating behavioural intention into action. If the individual has high self-esteem, an internal locus of control and a positive self-concept then it is likely that they will be more successful in stopping smoking or losing weight. However if this is not the case then they may feel that they are not able to change due to reasons beyond their control (Ewles and Simnett 2003; Katz et al. 2000; Tones and Tilford 2001).

Finally there are physical, cultural and socio-economic barriers and facilitating factors to consider with this model.

- We need to explore the factors that would support change and those that would not, for example, do individuals have the necessary knowledge and skills, e.g. cookery skills?

- Do they have communication skills, for example, are they able to explain to peers that their intention is to lose weight, stop smoking, do more exercise, and stop abusing drugs?

- Do they have self-regulatory skills? Are they able to monitor their diet and assess the effects on weight? Are they able to avoid temptation and reward themselves for successful health-related behavioural change?

Case scenario 1: Emily

Before we can apply this model to Emily, it is again necessary to consider the reasons that have led to her behaviour.

Emily is still very young, therefore we need to include her mother as well. Although she is one of the heaviest in the class she is not the only child who is overweight. There are pressures to consider related to bringing up two children as a single parent and there may also be a financial concern, which is why her mother may resort to cheap food which can be high in saturated fats and carbohydrates. Additionally technology has developed over the years and has led to a change in childhood activities which do not necessarily support healthy behaviour.

Application to practice

Compared with the Stages of Change Model and Health Belief Model, the Health Action Model may at first glance appear complex. This model helps us to explain *how* an individual makes the decision to change their health-related behaviour and what influences the outcome.

Case scenario 1: Emily

The teachers and school nurse have already involved Emily's mother. She recognizes that she is overweight and so she has designed an action plan with the school nurse. We can therefore assume that she has the behavioural intention and has made the decision to translate this into action by helping Emily and Josh to lose weight.

However, there are a number of factors that we need to deliberate about that may impact on whether Emily does lose weight and whether Josh is able to maintain a BMI within the normal range.

Belief system

- Does Emily's mother, Karen, understand the importance of weight loss from a factual perspective?

- Does Karen understand the link between the food she buys and her children's weight gain?

Motivation system

• Does Karen believe that it will make a difference to her children's overall health and well-being?

Normative system

• Is it the norm in Karen's family for everyone to be overweight?

• Is it the norm in Emily's class for the children to prefer watching TV or playing computer games rather than engaging in physical exercise?

The answers to these questions will affect whether Emily's mother's intention for her children to have a BMI within the normal range is translated into action. A combination of these factors may affect Emily's mother's intention to action the health promotion activities.

Personality factors: self-concept and self-esteem

• Emily's mother is a single parent with two small children. Her self-image and confidence may be low and therefore she gives into her children because they like the food she is cooking. We cannot assume that this is the case.

• If her self-concept is negative and if she does have low self-esteem then she may not be motivated to buy healthier food if she can afford to or to change the way she cooks.

Barriers to change: knowledge and skills

• Emily is choosy about the food she will eat and therefore could be challenging in her relationship with her mother. As a single parent Karen does not have anyone to support her if she decides to change her children's diets.

- Emily does not like to exercise, and prefers to watch TV or play on her computer.

- As her mother has limited cooking skills and provides food high in saturated fats and carbohydrates Emily may not understand the impact on her health. Six-year-olds are much more interested in 'play' and unlikely to consider their health at this point in their lives.

- Emily's mother can only afford to buy cheap food and therefore may feel that food high in carbohydrates is more filling, for example, chips.

- Being a single mother and living in rented accommodation with two small children could be stressful.

So, although Emily's mother has identified an action plan with the school nurse, the barriers suggested above could prevent her translating her behavioural intention into action and achieving behavioural change related to diet and exercise within the family.

Facilitating factors: knowledge and skills

- Emily's class teacher is concerned about the children's lack of knowledge about food and has asked the school nurse to help design a primary health promotion project on healthy diet and exercise for the children and their families.

- The school nurse has helped Emily's mother to prepare an action plan.

- Therefore it can be assumed that the relationship between the school and children's families is facilitative.

Possible health promotion activities

- Cookery demonstrations arranged by the school.
- Sports activities at the local sports centre for the whole family.

- Development of sport within Emily's school.

- Raising awareness through health education on the relationship between diet, exercise, weight and health.

- Emily and her class mates could design a poster illustrating how diet and exercise can benefit their health.

- The school curriculum could include more activities such as those suggested in Chapter 2 (see p. 39).

- Emily's mother could be referred to a community health promotion programme in which she is supported to develop her own skills. A number of UK community health promotion programmes were highlighted in Chapter 2, but an example specific to Emily's case is MEND 5–7. (For more information see http://mendcentral.org/MEND5–7.)

- This community health promotion programme could include activities that develop her assertiveness, self-esteem and confidence, and activities that would enable her to communicate and be more assertive, such as role play.

- Activities could also help her to develop her knowledge and skills, for example, developing her understanding of healthy menus and her cooking skills (psychomotor skills).

Self-regulatory skills are also important. Emily's mother could be encouraged to keep a diary of the family's diet and exercise habits. As with David, it would be important to explore the trends in their diet and explore the triggers that lead to her resorting to buying food that is cheap, high in saturated fats and carbohydrates and quick to cook.

Table 3.4 offers a critique of the Health Action model, outlining its advantages and disadvantages.

Table 3.4 Critique of the Health Action Model

Advantages	Disadvantages
Provides a framework to guide our thinking	Complex to understand
Acknowledges that there are barriers to change as well as facilitating factors, e.g. psychosocial and environmental factors	Limited evidence published of effectiveness
	Evidence suggests that it could be a disadvantage to only focus on the aspects that lead to behavioural choices
Identifies that health promotion work must include more than just health education	
Can be used to analyse whether the health promotion activity is likely to have an impact on an individual's behaviour	
Helps to explain what influences someone to change	
It considers all aspects including the wider determinants of health	

Source: Tones (1987); Hubley and Copeman (2008); Naidoo and Willls (2009)

Activity

- Compare and contrast the three models discussed in this chapter.

- Is there one particular model that would help you to think of health promotion activities to use with individuals you work with?

- Reflect on the reasons for your choice.

You may also like to consider other behavioural change models:

1 Beattie's model (1993, cited in Naidoo and Wills 2009) helps us to understand the political philosophy that underpins health promotion activity.

2 Tannahill's model of health promotion (Downie et al. 1996, cited in Naidoo and Wills 2009) explores how health education, health protection and prevention interconnectedness can facilitate health promotion work.

3   The Theory of Reasoned Action (Fishbein and Ajzen 1975, cited in Hubley and Copeman 2008) is similar to the Health Belief Model in that it explores beliefs and expectations. This model has been used in a variety of programmes such as exercise promotion (Rivis and Sheeran 2003).

Chapter summary

This chapter illustrates how The Stages of Change, Health Belief and Health Action health promotion models can help us to understand how individuals might make the decision to change their health-related behaviour. If those engaged in health promotion activity are aware of a number of health promotion models then they can compare and contrast them and choose the most appropriate model to guide their decision making for each individual or group of individuals. The choice of model will also depend on the individual's culture, personal values, beliefs and socio-economic and environmental status.

Implications for practice

• Understanding models and their application helps us to make informed decisions.

• Models help us to empower individuals to change as opposed to persuading or coercing them.

• Models provide us with an evidence-based framework for action.

Key points

• Health promotion models guide our practice and help us to explore factors that impact on successful behavioural change.

• Motivational interviewing helps us to develop our skills in exploring reasons for behaviour change (or not) in a structured way.

End of chapter questions

1   If you were working with an individual whose family were all overweight who wanted to eat healthily and do some exercise, which model would guide your thinking and help you to choose appropriate health promotion activities?

2   Having examined the strengths and limitations of the three models, does one offer more scope for use than the others?

3   Can you think of an occasion when motivational interviewing would have helped you to explore someone's readiness to change?

References

Abraham, C., Connor, M., Jones, F. and O'Connor, D. (2008) *Health Psychology*. London: Hodder Education.

Anderson, S., Keller, C. and McGowan, N. (1999) Smoking cessation: the state of science. The utility of the transtheoretical model in guiding interventions in smoking cessation. *Journal of Knowledge Synthesis for Nurses*, 6 (9).

Bandura, A. (2004) Health promotion by social and cognitive means. *Health Education and Behaviour*, April: 142–64.

Bundy, A. (2004) One essential direction: information literacy, information fluency. *Journal of e-Literacy*, 1 (1): 7–22.

Davies, M. and Macdowall, W. (2006) *Health Promotion Theory*. Maidenhead: Open University Press.

Ewles, L. and Simnett, I. (2003) *Promoting Health: A Practical Guide*, 5th edn. Edinburgh: Ballière Tindall.

Goodman-Brown, J. and Gottwald, M. (2008) Public health interventions. In J. Mitcheson (ed.) *Public Health Approaches to Practice*. Cheltenham: Nelson Thornes.

Green, J. and Tones, K. (2010) *Health Promotion: Planning and Strategies*. London: Sage.

Hillsdon, M. (2006) Motivational interviewing in health promotion. In W. Macdowall, C. Bonell and M. Davies (eds) *Health Promotion Practice*. Maidenhead: Open University Press.

Hubley, J. and Copeman, J. (2008) *Practical Health Promotion*. Cambridge: Polity.

Katz, J., Peberdy, A. and Douglas, J. (2000) *Promoting Health, Knowledge and Practice*. London: Open University Press in association with Palgrave.

Miller, W. and Rollnick, S. (2002) *Motivational Interviewing: Preparing People to Change*. New York: Guilford Press.

Naidoo, J. and Wills, J. (2009) *Public Health and Health Promotion Practice: Foundations for Health Promotion*. London: Baillière Tindall Elsevier.

NICE (2006) *Public Health Intervention Guidance – Brief Interventions and Referral for Smoking Cessation in Primary Care and Other Settings*. London: HMSO.

Pender, N., Murdaugh, C. and Parsons, M. (2010) *Health Promotion in Nursing Practice*, 6th edn. Upper Saddle River, NJ: Pearson.

Prochaska, J. and DiClemente, C. (1982) Transtheoretical therapy: towards a more inte-grateive model of change. *Psychotherapy: Theory Reserach and Practice*, 19: 276–88.

Prochaska, J. and DiClimente, C. (1984) *The Transtheoretical Approach: Crossing Traditional Boundaries of Therapy*. Harewood, IL: Dow-Jones.

Prochaska, J., DiClemente, C. and Norcross, J. (1992) In search of how people change: applications to addictive behaviours. *American Psychologist*, 47: 1102–14.

Registered Nurses Association of Ontario (2007) *Nursing Best Practice Guideline, Shaping the Future of Nursing. Integrating Smoking Cessation into Daily Nursing Practice*. Ontario: RNAO.

Rimmer, B. and Glanz, K. (2005) *Theory at a Glance: A Guide for Health Promotion Practice*, 2nd edn. Washington, DC: Department of Health and Human Services.

Rivis, A. and Sheeran, P. (2003) Social influences and the the theory of planned behaviour: evidence for a direct relationship between prototypes and young people's exercise behaviour. *Psychology and Health*, 18: 567–83.

Scriven, A. (2010) *Promoting Health: A Practical Guide*. London: Baillière Tindall Elsevier.

Tones, K. (1987) Devising strategies for preventing drug misuse: the role of the Health Action Model. *Health Education Research. Theory and Practice*, 2 (4): 305–17.

Tones, K. and Tilford, S. (2001) *Health Promotion: Effectiveness, Efficiency and Equity*. Cheltenham: Nelson Thornes.

West, R. (2005) Time for a change: putting the Transtheoretical (Stages of Change) Model to rest (editorial). *Addiction*, 100 (8): 1036–9.

Useful resources

Department of Health (2009) *Smoking Cessation Information Kit*. Hong Kong: DH, Tobacco Control Office.

NICE (2008) *NICE Public Health Guidance 10. Smoking Cessation Services in Primary Care, Pharmacies, Local Authorities and Workplaces, Particularly for Manual Working Groups, Pregnant Women and Hard to Reach Communities*. London: NICE.

Registered Nurses Association of Ontario (2007) *Nursing Best Practice Guideline, Shaping the Future of Nursing. Integrating Smoking Cessation into Daily Nursing Practice*. Ontario: RNAO.

4

Developing Self-Awareness
Jane Goodman-Brown

Introduction

This chapter focuses on individual self-awareness, as this is a prerequisite for empowerment, which will be discussed in the next chapter. The chapter begins by considering ways of developing self-awareness for ourselves as practitioners and for clients. One way of achieving this is through using the Johari window (Luft and Ingham 1969, cited in Rungapadiachy 1999). The chapter goes onto explore attitudes and behaviours with regard to health, and the notion of locus of control. The value that is placed on health is then discussed, and linked to Antonovsky's (1996) view of health and the importance of a sense of coherence, and the effect this has on health. Understanding the difference between health and illness in this context helps us to see why some individuals value their health and others do not. The chapter then examines the concepts of self-esteem and self-efficacy and links these to Bandura's (1986) theory of social learning. Finally the chapter will consider confidence and advocacy.

This book is focused on practical health promotion, but if we understand and can apply relevant theories this helps to give our practical ideas a sound foundation.

Learning objectives

By the end of this chapter the reader will be better able to:

- Understand the role of individual attitudes and behaviours, in relation to health

- Recognize why values are central to health promotion work, through exploring Antonovsky's theory

- Understand the pivotal role of self-esteem and self-efficacy in health promotion, and how to develop these

- Understand the role of confidence

- Recognize and explain the role of advocates and advocacy

- Apply ideas to practice

Developing self-awareness

Health, as we have established, is an individual concept and our attitudes towards it are influenced by our experiences. One of the important areas for exploration in relation to improving health is in developing our own self-awareness; part of this is being aware of our own values, attitudes and beliefs, as these all influence what we do. Basically, we have to get to know ourselves, and this chapter considers areas that we need to examine and links them to the case studies. In this chapter the main focus will be on two of the case studies: Hamed and Richard.

Becoming self-aware can be challenging and one way of overcoming this is to use tools such as the Johari window (see Figure 4.1).

The Johari window is a simple framework for developing our own self-awareness. It was devised by **Jo**seph Luft and **Har**ry Ingram and was originally intended for use with teams to consider what they know about each other, a

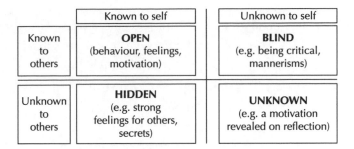

	Known to self	Unknown to self
Known to others	**OPEN** (behaviour, feelings, motivation)	**BLIND** (e.g. being critical, mannerisms)
Unknown to others	**HIDDEN** (e.g. strong feelings for others, secrets)	**UNKNOWN** (e.g. a motivation revealed on reflection)

Figure 4.1 A tool for developing self-awareness: the Johari window
Source: Luft and Ingham (1969, in Rungapadiachy, 1999). This figure was published in *Interpersonal Communication and Psychology for Health Care*, Rungapadiachy, Copyright Elsevier (1999)

problem or a situation. By exploring what is known it was hoped that communication would improve. It is also a useful framework or tool for individuals to think about their self and what they know about their own attributes.

It consists of four quadrants, and suggests that these quadrants reflect different dimensions of ourselves. The first quadrant is what we are aware of about our self (open); and the second what others know about us but we may not be aware of (blind). The third quadrant is what we know about ourselves but hide from others (hidden), i.e. any secrets we might have; and the final one is unknown to ourselves and to others (unknown). The aim of using this tool is to increase the open section through self-disclosure and to decrease all of the others. A small open window suggests that communication is poor, whereas a larger one indicates trust. However, disclosure should not be forced and sensitivity is essential. This framework could be used by us as individuals to consider our own attitudes and help us to become more self-aware. It could also be used with clients. For an example see the links to Richard's case scenario below.

Case scenario 3: Richard

Richard could use the framework on his own or with a health promoter, to think about his attitude towards his drinking habits, and help him to develop his self-awareness.

He is open and identifies that he drinks 30 units a week. However we do not know if this is accurate, or whether he has any issues that he hides from others or whether he has any hidden motivation about his drinking.

His attitudes towards his drinking might be revealed though reflection and disclosure leading to a bigger open area as below:

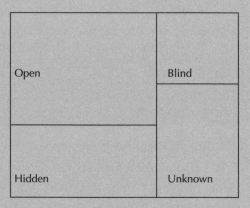

Here the open window is larger than the other quadrants, which would imply that the person is self-aware. If Richard could achieve this he might understand his behaviour and be willing to change.

Attitudes and behaviour

How we consider our health and that of others is influenced by our attitudes towards health and how we behave.

Attitudes

Attitudes do not always link to behaviour but they are relatively stable feelings towards an issue (Naidoo and Wills 2009). However changing attitudes may not lead to a change in behaviour. Attitudes combine knowledge and feelings about an issue and as a result are sometimes hard to change; attitudes can be influenced by information. They can also be influenced by success. Naidoo and Wills (2009) use the example of exercise to illustrate this point. Someone might be encouraged to take more exercise and change their attitude towards it by being given information, and by taking part and getting better at it so that it is enjoyable rather than a chore. As health promoters it is important that we are aware of the role of attitudes and success when encouraging individuals to try to change.

Green and Tones (2010) suggest one of the focuses of traditional health education is on attitude change and this is at odds with the theory of empowerment which is discussed in the next chapter. Here the focus is not on trying to change attitudes but on understanding the impact that an individual's attitudes will have on their behaviour.

Case scenario 2: Hamed

Hamed shows his attitude towards his diet and food when, during his consultation with the practice nurse, he wants to include Halima. This may not just be for support but also because he thinks that his diet and food are Halima's domain.

Behaviour

Understanding our behaviour and how it relates to our heath is one of the central ideas embedded in health promotion (Hubley and Copeman 2008). Behaviour refers to the 'specific acts that a person carries out' (Hubley and Copeman 2008: 62). There are a variety of types of behaviour that need to be considered in health promotion:

- **decision-based behaviour:** making a conscious decision, e.g. to eat healthily;
- **routine behaviour:** habit – perform regularly without thought, e.g. wearing a seat belt;
- **addictive behaviour:** reinforcement of the behaviour, either biologically or psychologically, e.g. smoking, alcohol;
- **behavioural norm:** behaviour shared by a group, e.g. an ethnic minority diet;

- **tradition:** behaviour passed down from one generation to the next, e.g. avoidance of a specific food.

(adapted from Hubley and Copeman 2008)

These types of behaviour overlap, for example, a decision to eat a particular diet due to a behavioural norm might become a habit. A group of young people might have a norm to practise safe sex following individual health promotion and this could then become a habit (Hubley and Copeman 2008).

Application to practice

> ## Case scenario 3: Richard's behaviour
>
> Some of Richard's behaviours appear to be as the result of addiction, e.g. smoking and drinking, as opposed to conscious decisions. Therefore he requires support to change these behaviours, but this will only be successful if he wants to change. Joining a support group might be helpful.
>
> However, his walking to work is a habit and this may have started out as a conscious decision. He needs to be supported to continue with this and maybe to build on it by taking more regular exercise. He could be helped with this by looking at his daily routine and identifying where more exercise could be included, for example walking to the shops at lunchtime to buy fresh food for his evening meal.

Perceived locus of control

Rotter (1966) suggested that an individual's perception of the amount of control they have over their life is an important factor in influencing their actions. He suggested that there are two approaches to individual control:

Internal locus of control: individuals with an internal locus of control think they are able to influence their lives and what happens to them through their behaviour. As a result of this they are more likely to take positive action to try and improve their life. For example if someone believes that they have a choice about whether or not they promote their own health through healthy eating they are more likely to try to eat healthily.

External locus of control: individuals with an external locus of control believe that nothing they do will influence their life. It is predetermined by fate or by powerful others and outside their control. As a result of this they are less likely to take action to try to change their situation. For example someone who has an external locus of control is less likely to try to change their diet for a healthy one as they may believe this will have no effect.

Application to practice

Case scenario 3: Richard

Richard would appear to have little interest in his health. He undertakes very few positive health-related actions. This may be because he feels that he has little control over his health, which would mean that he has an external locus of control. This may be exacerbated by his depression.

As a health promoter it would be important to discuss his attitude towards his health with him and find out his opinions, before trying to help him to improve his health.

Health locus of control

Further work on the concept of perceived locus of control was carried out by Kirscht (1972, cited in Green and Tones 2010). This focused on how locus of control specifically links to health and involved developing scales to measure individuals' locus of control in relation to their health. A range of research has since shown that health locus of control has poor predictive power with regard to behaviour change (Green and Tones 2010). However Walston and Walston (1982, cited in Green and Tones 2010) suggest that locus of control needs to be considered alongside other factors such as values and self-efficacy as discussed below.

Values

In the opening chapter we defined heath and discussed how one's view of health impacts on health and the value that is placed on it. Not everyone values health which makes the role of the health promoter more complex. However helping individuals to explore their perceptions of health might help them to identify the value they place on their health. Values, it must be remembered, are linked to emotions and help to determine what an individual thinks is important in their life (Naidoo and Wills 2009).

In Chapter 1, we discussed the WHO (1946: 5) definition that 'health is more than the absence of disease' and how this has changed perceptions of health, in that the approach to health is more holistic. For many, recognition of this might help to establish the value that individuals place on health. Over recent years there has been increasing emphasis on trying to understand how values influence health promotion and the way that it is approached.

Key point

Health is complex and our view is influenced by the value we place on it

One of the authors who has influenced our view of health is Aaron Antonovsky (1987, 1996). He suggests that rather than viewing health as the absence of disease or trying to prevent ill health by identifying risk factors, we should focus on looking at health and disease as a continuum and viewing everyone, whatever their risk factors, as having a place on this continuum. As health promoters we should try to ascertain what it is that enables some people to remain healthy despite their circumstances. Antonovsky (1996) suggests we should be interested in *why* and *how* an individual can be encouraged to participate in health-enhancing behaviours even though their health might be compromised.

Salutogenesis

Antonovsky (1987) purports that we should focus on salutogenesis – identifying what causes health as opposed to what causes disease. It is suggested that the focus is on people's resources and the capacity to create health (Green and Tones 2010). This links to the Ottawa Charter (WHO 1986) and the idea of strengthening the individual's health potential. He identifies that it can also link to groups and communities, but here our focus is on the individual. Antonovsky (1996) moves away from prevention as a result of risk factors to recognizing that life is stressful and we need to understand how to cope with stressors in such a way that we can improve health rather than try to prevent disease.

Kath and Pat

Kath is a 70-year-old woman who has a history of heart disease and is obese. She has followed the advice of the dietician and has changed her diet and lost weight and as a result her heart condition has improved.

Pat who is also 70 with a similar condition does not eat healthily and has not lost weight.

Salutogensis addresses why one person adopts a healthy behaviour and another does not. It is not focused on the risk factors or the external influences.

Generalized resistance resources

Antonovsky (1996) suggests that there are two main influences on health, the first of which is generalized resistance resources (GRR). These are individual material resources such as property and income or genetic and constitutional resources such as social support, intelligence, knowledge, identity and coping strategies, e.g. being flexible. The focus is not on the resources themselves but on the ability to use them to help the individual to move towards the health end of the continuum (Lindstom and Eriksson 2005).

Application to practice

Case scenario 2: Hamed

Hamed has generalized resistance resources (GRR) in the shape of a stable home with family support. His wife Halima has coping mechanisms to help him in that she can be flexible in her cooking to enable him to manage his diabetes. His GRR can be developed further by increasing his knowledge about diabetes and by helping him to develop his own coping strategies, possibly through group work and skills workshops in the local community centre.

Sense of coherence

According to Antonovsky (1987, 1996), the second main influence on health is developing a sense of coherence (SOC). Antonovsky identifies a sense of coherence as containing a sense of confidence that one's internal and external environment are predictable and that there is a high probability that things will turn out as well as can be expected. He suggests that those with a high sense of coherence can be helped to move towards the health end of the continuum, whatever their situation. A sense of coherence indicates internal and external environments that are structured, predictable and explicable, where resources are available to meet demands and challenges are worthy of investment and exchange. There is help available to cope with any stress (Green and Tones 2010). There are three main elements to a sense of coherence, which when individuals are confronted with a stressor helps them to cope:

> **Key point**
>
> Those with a high sense of coherence are more likely to be able to be helped to be healthy

1 Comprehensibility: they understand the challenge.

2 Manageability: they believe that the resources to cope with the challenge are available.

3 Meaningfulness: they want to be motivated to cope with the challenge.

Antonovsky (1996) indicates that these elements link to three of our value systems:

1 cognitive system – in that we understand the challenges of the issue;

2 behavioural system – in that we can act to change the situation;

3 motivational system – in that they have meaning for us.

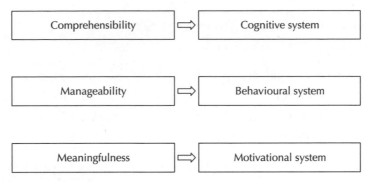

Figure 4.2 Sense of coherence

Antonovsky (1996) suggests the three factors included in a sense of coherence make the construct different and more comprehensive than other explanations of how we cope with change (see Figure 4.2).

Bruscia et al. (2008) indicate that because a sense of coherence impacts on these three systems it is important that health promotion activities address the three areas too. Therefore health promotion activities need to combine cognitive, emotional and social support. For example, to be effective, a smoking cessation programme needs to give information and ensure that it is understood but also needs to offer support to individuals. These ideas link to health literacy as discussed in the next chapter.

Application to practice

Case scenario 2: Hamed

Being diagnosed as a diabetic is a stressor for Hamed. This approach to health promotion does not emphasize preventing Hamed developing further complications. Instead the emphasis is on Hamed developing his health potential through utilizing his sense of coherence.

Comprehensibility needs to be addressed through health education on an individual or group basis. It is important the health education takes note of what Hamed already knows and builds on this. For example including discussions and debates to explore ideas in relation to *coping* with diabetes rather than health education talks.

Manageability can be emphasized by helping him identify resources and support groups both in the surgery and in the community. Community groups might be able to help him address any cultural issues such as help with adapting traditional menus.

Meaningfulness links to helping Hamed to identify how he can help himself and helping him to be motivated. This might be through access to a support group where he can see how others cope. It might also include offering him and his family regular follow-up and support.

Furthermore Antonovsky (1996) postulates that having a strong sense of coherence is influenced by life experience. He suggests the following:

- **Consistency** – Life experience is important. If an individual has had life experiences which are positive and which they can understand and predict, then their sense of coherence will be stronger.

- **Underload–overload balance** Life experiences that have utilized the individual's capabilities are conducive to improving the sense of coherence. If the life experiences have been challenging and the individual is unable to cope this has a negative impact on their sense of coherence.

- **Participation in decision making** is also seen as vital, in that individuals need to be active and participate in socially valued decision making rather than be controlled. It is suggested that this can be in relation to any aspect of life and not just health.

If individuals have life experiences that demonstrate these three factors they will have a strong sense of coherence. Initially it was suggested by Antonovsky (1996) that sense of coherence was the product of early life experience during the first three decades; it has now been suggested that there is some room for development in later life (Lindstrom and Eriksson 2006). Recognizing the possibility of development is important for health promotion as this can enable health promoters to help people to develop self-awareness with regard to their health.

Application to practice

Case scenario 2: Hamed

- **Consistency** is important for Hamed's family. They are supportive of each other and they have coped with other challenges such as adapting to a new culture while still relating to the important elements of their original culture. It is important that, as health promoters, we are consistent in our interactions with the family.

- **Balance** Hamed and his family have adapted and managed to retain balance in what they can cope with, but as health promoters it is our role to monitor the challenges and stressors and offer support.

- **Decision making** Is it important though to allow Hamed and his family to make their own decisions. Therefore as a health promoter, we need to identify resources and enable Hamed and his family to make choices and retain control.

Sense of coherence can be measured by a self-report scale and Antonovsky (1993) developed two well known ones. Research suggests that rating oneself highly links to a higher sense of coherence and demonstrates a better quality of life (Erikson and Lindstrom 2007).

Antonovsky (1996) goes on to suggest that because coherence is individual, it is applicable whatever the culture of the individual. Lindstrom and Eriksson (2006) state that there is a range of evidence since the 1980s to support this.

Application to practice

Considering salutogensis has enabled us to look at health promotion from a different perspective. It has helped us to see which activities are relevant and to understand why we use them to develop an individual's self-awareness.

Self-esteem and self-efficacy

These two important concepts link to knowledge of self; they are also part of Bandura's social learning theory and were first introduced in Chapter 3 when we discussed the Heath Action Model.

Bandura (1986) proposes that we all learn through experience and by observing others. He suggests that learning is the result of interaction between the individual and the environment. The individual is influenced by their beliefs about their self. Another important aspect of social learning theory is the role of modelling. This theory suggests that we model ourselves on others. This can be positive and is why some health promoters use celebrities to endorse healthy behaviour but it can also be negative as people may try to emulate a hero who does not necessarily behave well.

Stop and think

Can you think of examples when a celebrity has been used effectively to support a healthy lifestyle behaviour change?

Overall social learning theory is relevant to health promotion because it emphasizes the importance of understanding individuals within their social context (Hubley and Copeman 2008).

Self-esteem

Self-esteem is how an individual feels about themselves; whether or not they think they are of value. Low self-esteem often means that individuals are critical of their self and their abilities. It has been suggested that those with low self-esteem are more likely to be involved in negative health behaviours whereas those with high self-esteem are more able to resist pressure. Those with low self-esteem often doubt their self and this may mean that they find it difficult to communicate with others and to meet their own needs. In health promotion one of the roles of the

Key point

Self-esteem is about how you feel about yourself

health promoter is to enable individuals to develop their self-esteem and Scriven (2010: 136) suggests that one way to do this is:

- to be aware of the client's feelings;

- to use opportunities to help clients learn how to deal with difficult feelings;

- to listen to the feelings and acknowledge that most people have the same difficult feelings;

- to label the feelings;

- to set limits and identify strategies for dealing with the problem.

Some health promoters suggest that enhancing self-esteem is a health promotion goal in its own right and does not need to be linked to any particular situation (Hubley and Copeman 2008). Rather, it should be at the heart of everything we do.

Stop and think

Can you think of an incident in your practice when helping someone to develop their self-esteem has been an important part of helping them improve their health?

Application to practice

Case scenario 3: Richard

Practical ways of developing self-esteem

Richard would appear to be have low self-esteem; he can't be bothered to cook and has little time for relaxation or a social life. As a health promoter working with Richard, it is important to explore how he feels about himself and his life.

> You could do this by asking him to list the positive and negative aspects of himself and then try to turn some of the negatives into positives. For example he might state that he is easily bored. A positive for this is that he might like new challenges. Or he might state that he wants to have more rest. Acknowledging this is important and not being lazy, and might help him to change his perception of his behaviour and help him to begin to develop higher self-esteem.

Self-efficacy

Self-efficacy is possibly one of the most important prerequisites for behaviour change. It is defined as the extent to which the behaviour can be achieved by an individual and their belief in their self (Abraham et al. 2008). Basically this means whether or not an individual believes that they can change and it differs from self-esteem in that it is situation-specific not a general feeling (Davies and Macdowall 2006). For example, if someone

> **Key point**
>
> Self-efficacy is about self-belief

intends to give up smoking but they don't think that they will be able to achieve this, their chances of success are slim. However if they have a strong self-belief and think that they will be successful then they are more likely to be successful. They may not have high self-efficacy in other aspects of their lives but still may be successful in stopping smoking. This concept links to empowerment as discussed in the next chapter and to locus of control, which is discussed above.

Self-efficacy can be enhanced through:

- observational learning and participatory learning – by identifying others who have been successful at changing an aspect of their behaviour an individual might be able to change too, for example, through a support group.

- verbal persuasion – explanations about why they might be successful could help; however this must link to empowerment and giving enough information so that they make an informed choice.

- perception of psychological and affective states – discussion about how they feel about the proposed change and the likelihood of them being successful, as well as listening to their responses before making joint decisions. This may be achieved through individual counselling and active listening (Abraham et al. 2008; Davies and Macdowall 2006).

Application to practice

Case scenario 3: Richard

Richard appears to have limited self-efficacy. He eats an unbalanced diet and he smokes and drinks to excess. We do not know if he would be prepared to change any of these behaviours.

It is important to establish with him which of these behaviours he would like to change and which he feels he might be most successful at changing.

If he wants to stop smoking, observational and participatory learning could be utilized by encouraging him to join a smoking cessation group where others have been successful.

Although health promotion is not about persuasion, giving him information might help him to feel that he is able to succeed. It is also important to explore with Richard how he feels about the issue and to encourage him to make his own decisions rather than telling him what to do. He can make a decision using a decisional balance matrix and all of this will help him to feel that he is able to change.

Self-confidence

Developing self-confidence is an important aspect of becoming self-aware. Without confidence it is unlikely that an individual will be able to change or have the desire to change. Having confidence can help in making accurate decisions. Confidence is about recognizing individual strengths and areas for development and

Key point

Self-confidence is essential in decision making and awareness raising

being able to utilize these fully. For the individual this is enhanced by recognizing their achievements and encouraging them to continue to develop and grow. It requires the health promoter to give accurate information and help the individual to develop their skills. Success will help to breed self-confidence and enable people to make relevant decisions.

Barr and Hashagan (2000) developed 'The Building Blocks of Community Development' and in this they suggest that in order to help communities develop individuals need to have increased self-confidence, and this is achieved by health promoters encouraging and promoting individual confidence through the use of accurate information and empowerment.

Application to practice

Case scenario 2: Hamed

Hamed lacks confidence in his own abilities to make decisions about how he can improve his health. He can be supported through addressing his information needs with culturally appropriate information and by being referred to a community support group. He is also encouraged by Halima's involvement in his care. Recognition of successful changes will help to develop his confidence as will helping him to make logical decisions about his actions, for example using a decisional balance tool – making a list of the advantages and disadvantages of making a change to his diet to improve his diabetes control.

Advantages	Disadvantages
• reduce risks of diabetic complications	• having to give up some foods he enjoys
• feel better	• change eating habits
• less tired, more energy for family and work commitments	• need to learn new cooking skills
• lose weight	
• improve family health	

The final aspect to be considered in this chapter is advocacy. In order to develop self-awareness and improve health and well-being there is a need for individuals to become advocates for their own health needs. As health promoters we also need to be aware of our role as advocates for clients.

Advocacy

Advocacy links to the Ottawa Charter (WHO 1986) where it is suggested that being an advocate is one of the three main prerequisites for improving health. Advocates should represent disadvantaged groups and lobby for policy change to support these groups. The role of an advocate is to encourage debate and support change and this is achieved through reframing issues so that they are relevant to individuals and to policy makers (Green and Tones 2010).

Advocacy links to self-awareness and to community development. As professionals we need not only to help our clients to develop their self-awareness but we need to develop our own self-awareness in order to support them. Professionals can act as an advocate for a group or for an individual but to be successful they should ensure that they:

> **Key point**
>
> Advocates can work with individuals or groups

1   Set an agenda for the change: identify what the issue is and who is affected by it

2   Make the issue relevant to the public: although the client group or individual might be clear what change is required, in order to lobby for change it must be relevant to the public too

3   Advocate specific solutions: requesting change without having ideas for solutions will be ineffective

(Baum 2001, cited in Tones and Green 2004).

In order to achieve these three things the health promoter needs to be self-aware and have established with the client group or individual what their needs are and what is required to help them to achieve these needs. Advocacy is not about professionals trying to meet their own agenda; instead it requires them to support the client's agenda. Clients may also want to be advocates for their own needs, and user groups such as Diabetes UK and the British Heart Foundation, are very successful at advocating for the needs of their members.

Application to practice

Case scenario 3: Richard

As an individual Richard might need the support of an advocate in helping him adjust to his changed health status. As he is employed it might be important that he is supported to continue working.

Baum's (2001) suggestions can help with planning the approach that an advocate could take.

1   Richard may need help to decide what his agenda at work is and may need to consider whether he wants to return full-time or part-time.

2   He needs to explore with his employer what the benefits of him returning to work might be.

3   He also needs to think about clear solutions which identify ways that he could possibly work part-time to reduce his stress.

For an individual to be an advocate for their own needs they have to be clear what the issues that affect them are, so they may require help from professionals to clarify these issues. We can help by offering accurate information and enabling them to present the ideas in an appropriate format.

Chapter summary

This chapter has explored the role of self-awareness in helping individuals to improve their health. Attitudes and behaviours are linked to Rotter's locus of control and this helps us to understand how people's attitudes towards change affect whether or not they can change. We have explored how Antonovsky's theory helps us to understand that values influence the individual's willingness to participate in health-enhancing behaviours. In the previous chapter we introduced self-esteem and self-efficacy as part of the Health Action Model and this chapter highlights how these concepts are pre-requisites for successful behavioural change. Finally this chapter explains the role that self-confidence and advocacy have in developing self-awareness and how this helps an individual with decision making and changing behaviour.

Implications for practice

- Self-awareness is complex but essential for change to occur, and everyone has different levels of self-awareness; therefore as health promoters it is imperative to identify individual levels, as well as our own.

- Understanding the theory behind self-awareness helps us to approach developing self-esteem, self-efficacy and self-confidence in a structured manner.

Key points

- Recognizing the breadth of factors that affect self-awareness will impact on our practice.

- Effective health promotion is underpinned by the relevant theory.

End of chapter questions

1   Are some types of behaviour more difficult to change than others?

2   What are the strengths and limitations of salutogenesis?

3   Why is it important to develop an individual's self-esteem, self-efficacy and self-confidence?

References

Abraham, C., Connor, M., Jones, F. and O'Connor, D. (2008) *Health Psychology*. London: Hodder Education.

Antonosky, A. (1987) *Unravelling the Mystery of Health*. San Francisco, CA: Jossey Bass.

Antonovsky, A. (1993) The structure and properties of the Sense of Coherence Scale. *Social Science Medicine*, 36(6): 725–33.

Antonovsky, A. (1996) The salutogenic model as a theory to guide health promotion. *Health Promotion International*, 11(1): 11–18.

Bandura, A. (1986) *Social Foundations of Thought and Action*. Englewood Cliffs, NJ: Prentice-Hall.

Barr, A. and Hashagen, S. (2000) *ABCD Handbook: A Framework for Evaluating Community Development*. London: CDF Publications.

Baum, F. (2001) Healthy public policy. In T. Heller, R. Muston, M. Siddell and C. Lloyd (eds) *Working for Health*. London: Sage.

Bruscia, K., Shultis, C. and Denney, K. (2008) The sense of coherence in hospitalised cancer patients. *Journal of Holistic Nursing*, 26(4): 289–94.

Dawies, M. and Macdowall, W. (2006) *Health Promotion Theory*. Maidenhead: Open University Press.

Eriksson, M. and Lindstrom, B. (2007) Antonovsky's Sense of Coherence Scale and its relation with quality of life: a systematic review. *Journal of Epidemiology and Community Health*, 61(11): 938–44.

Green, J. and Tones, K. (2010) *Health Promotion: Planning and Strategies*. London: Sage.

Hubley, J. and Copeman, J. (2008) *Practical Health Promotion*. Cambridge: Polity.

Lindstom, B. and Eriksson, M. (2006) Contextualising salutogenensis and Antonovsky in public health development. *Health Promotion International*, 23(3): 238–4.

Naidoo, J. and Wills, J. (2009) *Foundations for Health Promotion*. London: Baillière Tindall.

Rotter, J. (1966) Generalized expectancies for internal versus control of reinforcements. *Psychological Monographs*, 80: 609.

Rungapadiachy, D. (1999) *Interpersonal Communication and Psychology for Health Care*. Oxford: Butterworth Heinemann.

Soviven, A. (2010) *Promoting Health: A Pratical Guide*. London: Baillière Tindall Elsevier.

Tones, K. and Green, J. (2004) *Health Promotion: Planning and Strategies*. London: Sage.

WHO (World Health Organisation) (1946) *Constitution of the World Health Organisation*. www.who/int/governance/eb/who_constitution_en.pdf. (accessed 29 November 2011).

WHO (1986) *The Ottawa Charter*. http://www.who/int/hpr/NPH/docs/ottawa_charter_hp.pdf (accessed 29 November 2011).

5

Developing Skills
Mary Gottwald

Introduction

The last chapter considered a number of health promotion activities that could be used to develop self-awareness. One of the hardest aspects of health promotion work is the application of theory to practice, so this chapter will begin by discussing activities that will enable individuals and communities to feel more empowered and to take control of factors which influence their health. It will then continue by exploring a number of activities that could facilitate the development of know-ledge and skills, to directly influence health-related behaviours in relation to life skills such as assertiveness, communication and problem solving. Hamed (case scenario 2) and David (case scenario 4) will be used to illustrate the application of these activities.

Learning objectives

By the end of this chapter the reader will be better able to:

- Understand how health promotion activities could be used to empower individuals to make health-related decisions

- Understand how health promotion activities could enhance skills, in relation to assertiveness, communication and problem solving

- Identify and apply relevant activities to practice

Empowerment

In Chapter 1, health promotion was defined as 'the process of enabling people to increase control over and to improve their health' (WHO 1986: 1) and one way to achieve this is through empowering individuals and communities. According to Hubley and Copeman (2008: 252), an empowered individual is one 'who has the necessary information, skills and confidence to play an active role in their recovery'. Macdowall et al. (2006: 97) take this one step further by adding 'and opportunity to develop a sense of control and mastery over life circumstances'. Therefore as health promoters, we need to create supportive contexts that enable individuals and communities to feel empowered, and thus have improved life chances (Pendelton and Schultz-Krohn 2006; Thompson 2007). Thompson (2007: 41) summarizes a key aspect, i.e. 'empowerment is working with people rather than doing things to or for them'. Enablement and empowerment are not the same concepts but are interrelated. Enablement concerns the personal aspects that we discussed in Chapter 4, such as developing confidence and self-esteem and also includes the professionals identifying goals and supporting them to succeed in attainment of these goals.

Empowerment involves collaboration and working together, and deciding on goals and action plans, and therefore it is necessary that we ensure that health promotion activities engage the individual, so that they are 'enabled to empower themselves' (Thompson 2007: 22). Collaboration and working together is more likely to increase motivation and avoid

Key point

Collaboration facilitates empowerment

conflict. In order to achieve this we have to begin by establishing a rapport and for this we have to be able to communicate clearly, and be able to listen to what individuals are saying. Due to time constraints within our practice, it is generally not feasible to establish a *relationship*, as this takes time to develop, and therefore we have to aim to establish a *rapport* as this can be achieved reasonably quickly, providing we have the necessary skills such as listening to what individuals are telling us, as opposed to forging ahead with our own agenda and ideas (Thompson 2007).

Negotiation is also a requirement, as we must not tell individuals what to do, for example, say to David that he must give up abusing drugs or tell Hamed that he must exercise five times a week. Although negotiation is one of the first steps in establishing a rapport, we must also ensure that we do not agree to goals that we know are detrimental and inappropriate. It is therefore essential that we also demonstrate empathy and recognize how those we work with are feeling (Thompson 2007). Teamwork and networking supports both us and those we are working with, and ensures that resources provided meet the needs of both the individual and communities in which they live (Payne 2000).

Activity

Reflect on your own skills.

- Do you engage those you work with in order to establish a rapport?
- Do you negotiate action plans, while at the same time ensuring that decisions made are not detrimental and inappropriate?
- If your answer to these questions is 'yes', what evidence do you base this on?
- If your answer to either of these is 'no' or 'not sure', then consider how you could continue to develop your skills further.
- What support would you need from your manager?

At times in our practice our negotiation skills are not sufficient to resolve issues and conflict may arise.

- How do you resolve any conflict that arises?

Trust

A rapport will not be established if there is either conflict or a lack of trust. Individuals such as David and Richard may well have tried a number of times to stop abusing substances, such as cigarettes and drugs. However, if the support that they have been given has been disempowering or negative in any way, then there is likely to be a lack of trust and this in turn is likely to affect any partnership or achievement of behavioural change. Therefore in order to achieve a positive health outcome, we must establish rapport, build trust and avoid conflict.

Application to practice

Case scenario 2: Hamed

Hamed has put on quite a lot of weight, and his blood glucose level indicates that he may have diabetes type II. The nurse has given him some information about improving his diet, and therefore Hamed may begin to have the knowledge about the importance of changing his health-related behaviours. However, if he does not have assertiveness or communication skills, then he may not feel empowered to talk with Halima about the need to re-think her traditional cooking and he may not feel empowered to make the decision to do more exercise.

Hamed and Halima have shown that they are able to initially problem solve, as they utilized the free screening for diabetes. However, if they choose to go to the support group offered by the nurse, then health promoters would need to work with them by identifying possible strategies that will make them feel empowered. By working together and by including Hamed and Halima in decision making, their autonomy would thus be respected (Pendelton and Schultz-Krohn 2006).

Case scenario 4: David

David has signed up for a smoking cessation group, and is now taking part in a needle-exchange programme. The nurse has organized for him to work in the prison kitchen, and David has identified that he would also like to sign up for the new 'building respect and understanding' programme. David has also indicated that life outside prison is a great hardship.

We could assume that David will be given information in these programmes, and from the case scenario, we can see that he is being provided with opportunities to sign up for a variety of programmes. However, if this information does not take into consideration David's learning difficulties then it will be meaningless. In order to enable David to empower himself and make the decision to change his health-related behaviour, it would be important to discuss and negotiate his goals and strategies that would enable him to develop aspects of his life that he finds challenging. Providing opportunities to develop skills such as confidence, communication, assertiveness and self-esteem need to be considered.

Due to his learning disability, David may not recognize the strengths that he has; he also has a history of substance misuse, and these can affect the health-related decisions that he makes (Thompson 2007), therefore working in partnership and providing opportunities will facilitate empowerment.

Health education, as part of a health promotion programme would achieve this 'information giving' aspect through the provision of leaflets, health websites and DVDs. However, this does not mean that an individual would feel empowered to make the decision to change their health-related behaviour. In order to take behavioural change one step further, opportunities need to be provided to develop confidence (discussed in Chapter 4) in order for individuals to play an 'active role in their recovery'. 'Health literacy skills' would also have to be developed. Health literacy 'refers to the personal, cognitive and social skills, which determine the ability of individuals to gain access to, understand and use information to promote and maintain good health' (Nutbeam 2000: 263). So, leaflets on the importance of giving up smoking or leaflets on a healthy diet would give individuals access to this information.

> **Key point**
>
> Provision of leaflets alone does not necessarily empower an individual to make the decision to change

However, they also need to be given the opportunities to develop skills in assertiveness (to say 'no' when offered a cigarette for example) or the opportunity to develop cookery skills related to healthy menus.

In Chapter 3, we suggested that cookery demonstrations could be included in the school curriculum for Emily, her classmates and their parents. We also suggested that Emily's mother could be referred to a community health promotion programme, in which she is supported to develop her own skills. We have also discussed how schools in the UK have ceased to sell unhealthy foods, such as crisps and chocolate in vending machines, and how canteens provide healthy options to children. These activities could facilitate Emily and her mother to become more empowered.

So, we can see that there are three levels to developing the health literacy skills that are essential to empowerment, and these ideas are similar to salutogenesis discussed in Chapter 4:

1   Provision of information

2   In order to understand and use this information, opportunities to develop necessary practical skills such as communication, problem solving and assertiveness need to be provided to individuals. Confidence is also crucial in order that individuals can use these practical skills.

3   Organizational change is also required, so that social action to develop policies (e.g. within schools) can be achieved.

(Mogford et al. 2010; Nutbeam 2000)

Scriven (2005) also identifies three aspects to be considered when developing empowerment within individuals and communities:

1   developing self-esteem and self-efficacy;

2   developing awareness through health education;

3   developing life skills such as problem solving, communication and assertiveness.

This chapter will focus on developing the life skills identified in point 3.

Application to practice

Case scenario 2: Hamed

Halima notices a poster at the local surgery, which explains the signs and symptoms of diabetes and offers free screening. Clearly she has linked this information to Hamed, who is always thirsty and whose father was diagnosed with diabetes. The practice nurse provides some information and she goes through this to ensure Hamed understands; she also suggests he attends a support group for those newly diagnosed with diabetes. However, as we have discussed above, providing information is not enough to empower Hamed and Halima to make the decision to change their diets. They also need to be given opportunities to develop their skills in relation to preparing and cooking healthy meals.

Key points

Providing information is important but in order to feel empowered it is important to develop

1 self-esteem
2 self-efficacy
3 confidence

as well as the following life skills

1 problem solving
2 communication
3 assertiveness

Case scenario 4: David

David has recently signed up to join a smoking cessation group, and has been offered a place in a reading class to help him catch up with his lost schooling. Through health education, he may be provided with information on the benefits of stopping smoking, but unless this information is presented at a suitable level, David may not understand. He has also been offered a place on the detox programme, and so is receiving support in addition to information. Once David does understand about the benefits of giving up smoking, further health promotion activities could be included, e.g. increasing his self-awareness, self-esteem and self-efficacy and confidence (as discussed in the last chapter) and also his problem solving, communication and assertiveness skills.

Empowering ourselves

So far, we have discussed how we can enable individuals to empower themselves to make health-related changes. However, if we do not feel empowered ourselves, then it is not easy to empower others. We therefore must ensure that we are up to date with our practice and theories from health promotion. We also need to ensure that we have the support from managers to continue to develop our knowledge and skills and this in turn involves critical reflective thinking, to understand and identify our needs (Thompson 2007; Mullins 2010).

Keeping up to date with the evidence base of our practice and health promotion theories enables us to work in partnership. Using our knowledge and skills helps us to work with individuals to identify their health-related issues and to discuss possible courses of action and helps us to work with them to prioritize areas of change. It may feel as if we are not in control, but working together and establishing rapport and trust allows individuals to voice their concerns and feel involved in the negotiation process, and therefore they are more likely to engage in health promotion activities.

Communication

When we think about communication (see Figure 5.1) it is important to reflect on our own communication skills, as well as health promotion activities that could facilitate the development of communication skills within the individuals and communities with which we work. We have seen that health promotion is about empowering individuals to make the decision to change their health-related behaviour, and so it is essential when communicating with individuals and communities that we work in partnership, and enable autonomy and empowerment as opposed to making the decisions and being judgemental. Establishing trust and respecting individual ideas and values are also crucial to this partnership (Scriven 2010). Assertive communication means that we also have to express ourselves in an honest and clear manner; in other words, not using jargon, acronyms or language that is too complex or simple for the listener (Bishop 2010).

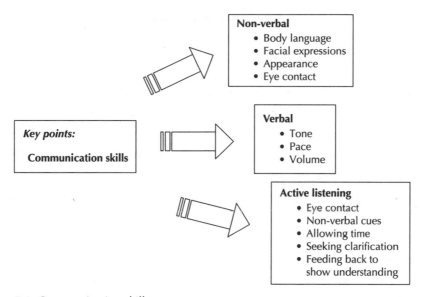

Figure 5.1 Communication skills
Source: Bishop (2010); Bond (2006); Hubley and Copeman (2008); Scriven (2010); Wills and Earle (2007)

Case scenario 2: Hamed

Telling Hamed that he is overweight and must lose weight is judgemental. Explaining that weight and lack of exercise can impact on diabetes is not.

Case scenario 4: David

Telling David that smoking is silly nowadays is being judgemental. Discussing the general benefits of not smoking is more likely to empower David to consider giving up smoking.

David has identified that he feels life outside the prison is a great hardship, so providing opportunities for David to talk through why he feels like this will help him to be more direct and assertive in his communications.

Non-verbal and verbal communication

Non-verbal and verbal communication are central to health promotion work, and are linked to values, self-esteem, self-efficacy and confidence as discussed in the last chapter. If individuals do not feel good about themselves, then the work of the health promoter will need to focus on developing self-esteem and self-efficacy, before developing communication skills. Communication is also linked to assert-iveness and problem solving, which will be discussed later in this chapter. Communication is not only concerned with the transmission of messages but also making sure that the message has been received and understood (Tones and Green 2004).

First of all we will consider communication from the health promoter's perspective. Non-verbal communication can be powerful, and therefore we need to think about our own body language, for example, use of facial expressions and gestures; our appearance (e.g. dressing too formally could be frightening, but dressing too casually could be considered rude). We should also consider the tone and pace of our voice because speaking too fast could be confusing, but speaking too slowly could be considered patronizing.

Active listening

We have to show that we are actively listening, as this helps individuals to feel included and more confident. This can be achieved through allowing time for individuals to reflect and think about what they want to say. We need to remember that 'silences' are okay; some eye contact is necessary; however, we also have to consider cultural aspects, as too much eye contact or too little eye contact can be considered rude (Bishop 2010). Asking for clarification demonstrates that we are listening, for example, asking Hamed what traditional cooking involves or asking David how he feels about joining the detox programme, as well as the smoking cessation programme. Finally we can feed back to individuals to show that we have heard and understood them, for instance by going through the main points they have discussed with us.

Gaining information

Another skill that is essential is to be able to gain information through questioning. Both open and closed questions are useful; however, we should be careful because closed questions tend to be answered with 'yes, no or maybe'. If more detailed information is required, open questions must be used.

Key point

Think about the kind of information you want to gather and then consider using open or closed questions

Case scenario 2: Hamed

Open questioning

'From what you have said to me, I understand that your wife is a good, traditional cook and that you enjoy her cooking. Could you tell me more about the meals that Halima prepares for you both?'

Case scenario 4: David

Open questioning

'You mentioned to me that you find life outside the prison a great hardship, and would like to make some changes. So that we can think about support once you are released, it would be useful to know what changes you would like to make.'

The first part of both these communications summarizes one of the key points that have been raised in initial discussions with Hamed and Halima and David and the second then asks for more information.

Giving information

The final skill to be considered is to be able to give information. Today there are numerous ways that health promoters can provide information, e.g. through

Table 5.1   Critique of information resources

	Advantages	*Disadvantages*
Leaflets	Individuals can read these in their own time and always have them to refer to.	Leaflets do not necessarily consider education level.
Posters	Can raise awareness.	Too much information may mean posters are not read.
DVDs	Health promoters can pause and allow time for questions and discussion.	Equipment is not always reliable and therefore other media are needed.
CDs	Useful for those whose learning style is supported through listening.	Difficult if learning style is visual.
Internet	Useful for providing a variety of information.	Reliability could be questioned.

Source: Scriven (2010)

leaflets, posters, DVDs, CDs, and individuals who have access to home computers or library computers can gain information from websites (Scriven 2010). There are advantages and disadvantages to each of these methods and careful consideration is necessary. Some examples are provided in Table 5.1.

Activity

Some advantages and disadvantages have been identified in Table 5.1

- Think of some further advantages and disadvantages.
- Which methods would be useful in your area of practice?

When we discussed health literacy skills earlier, we highlighted that giving information is not enough; we must make sure that individuals not only understand the information but are then given opportunities to develop the necessary skills that would empower them to successfully achieve behavioural change.

Application to practice

Case scenario 2: Hamed

Written information is provided, and the practice nurse goes through this with Hamed. However, it is important that the practice nurse selects appropriate leaflets or handouts; it is useful to use a mixture of written and visual presentation, and it is essential to ensure the language used is not too complex but not patronizing. We have also discussed that leaflets, DVDs or CDs are not necessarily sufficient and Hamed and Halima may like to utilize opportunities to develop healthy cooking skills, as well as understand more about exercise.

Communication would fail if they were just advised to take more exercise, so specific examples could be suggested, for example:

- Walk for 5 minutes at a comfortable pace
- Walk for 3 minutes at a slightly faster pace
- Walk for 5 minutes at a comfortable pace
- Do this 3 times for the first week

Then for the next 2 weeks:

- Walk for 10 minutes at a comfortable pace
- Walk for 5 minutes at a faster pace
- Walk for 10 minutes at a comfortable pace

Key points

Give specific examples of activities

Set achievable SMART goals

Case scenario 4: David

Similarly David could be given information via leaflets, handouts, DVDs and CDs. As he is joining a detox programme and smoking cessation programme, he may also be given information via PowerPoint presentations and flip charts.

Key point

Use different methods when providing information

As stated previously, David has a number of health-related behavioural changes that he is considering, and so it is important for the prison staff to collaborate in relation to the amount of information David is being given.

As he has learning difficulties, there is also a need to consider the level of information, because if too complex then David could lose confidence and his self-esteem could be affected. If PowerPoint presentations are part of these programmes, then also providing David with appropriate leaflets or DVDs would ensure that he is given the opportunity to read and listen at his own pace. Including him in the programmes provides him with opportunities to talk with peers and prison staff so he would not feel that he is alone in making these health-related choices and changes.

Barriers to communication

Before we can think about health promotion activities that would enhance the communication skills in those with whom we work there are barriers that need to be considered, some of which are listed below:

Context

- Are you using a private, quiet room?
- Is the room too warm or too cold?
- Have you thought about the layout of the room?
- Does the individual have their hearing aid switched on?

Language

- Are you using health and/or social care jargon?
- Is English their first language?
- Are you using the right level of English?

- Are you listening to how things are being said?

- Are you providing too much information to remember?

- Are you giving specific examples?

- Are you giving the same message as others in the team?

- Are you communicating as the expert or are you working in partnership with the individual?

Emotions

- Is pain, stress, anxiety, anger, denial apparent?

(adapted from Ewles and Simnett 2003)

Activity

- If you answer 'no' to any of the questions above, then it would be important that you reflect on what changes you could make in the future.

- Reflect on your own practice, and consider whether there are other barriers to communication.

- Could you develop your communication skills further?

- What support do you need to do this?

- Could you discuss this with your line manager or other colleagues?

Principles

Before we move on to think about how individual communication skills can be facilitated, so that successful behavioural changes can be achieved, there are some fundamental principles to be considered.

Communication is an interactive and reciprocal process, and therefore it is important to:

- establish mutual common ground

- reduce uncertainties that can block communication

- think in terms of outcomes

- demonstrate flexibility

(Silverman et al. 2005)

Application to practice

Case scenario 4: David

David receives health services within the prison system, and is part of a programme to combine health care with rehabilitation and resettlement on discharge. David also has learning difficulties and has a low level ability in relation to reading.

This programme will involve David working alongside other prisoners, prison staff and support services on his release, so he will be communicating with a number of different individuals either on a one-to-one basis and/or within a group.

Suggested health promotion activities (one-to-one)

- Cognitive behavioural one-to-one skills training, to help David think about situations, his thoughts, feelings and actions. Does he find communicating his ideas and needs to others difficult? In what particular situations does he find communicating difficult? (Westbrook et al. 2008)

- Getting David to think about his posture, eye contact, facial expressions, tone, volume and pace of voice.

- Practising scenarios, for example, first of all engaging David in talking about something that he enjoys. This can help him to relax while developing his confidence.

- Role playing, for example, David's first meeting with support services on discharge; getting him to practise talking about the support that he needs. After the role play, it is important to allow time for David to

---

reflect on the role play, as well as his non-verbal communication, tone, volume and pace of voice.

Group activities

- Before any group work can be undertaken, trust needs to be established within the group. Getting the group to work within small groups to identify ground rules will begin to establish this trust and once agreed, a flip chart can be used to collate suggested ground rules.

- Ice breakers are also effective, as we cannot assume everyone in the group knows each other.

> **Key points**
>
> Agree 'ground rules'
> Lead the ice breaker activity in an enthusiastic manner
> Ice breakers are short activities
> (Knox 2011)

- Working within small groups encourages participation, for instance, sharing strategies in relation to smoking and drug cessation within small group discussion; listing three or four strategies that have worked; getting one person from each group to feed back their strategies. This enables individuals to share experiences in a safe environment.

- Showing that you care and are working in partnership can make a difference (Payne 2000); letting the group know that all contributions are valuable will continue to establish the trust within the group. This can be achieved through active listening and valuing ideas.

Possible ice breakers

1   Date of birth and introductions

- Get everyone to line themselves up in relation to their date of birth.

- Then in groups of three, ask each other to introduce themselves.

- After five minutes ask each group of three to introduce each other to the whole group.

2   True or false.

- Ask each person to write down one true fact and two false facts about themselves and then read them out.

- The group votes which is true and which are false.

3   Interview

- Divide the group into pairs and ask the pairs to introduce themselves and then talk with each other to identify two facts, e.g. one hobby and one 'wish' (two minutes each).

- Bring the group back together and get each person to present these facts about their partner.

(Knox 2011)

Assertiveness

Assertiveness does not mean communicating what you want in a passive or aggressive manner or communicating in a manipulative manner; it means being able to express your thoughts confidently, plainly and explicitly (Bishop 2010; Hubley and Copeman 2008; Scriven 2010). Assertiveness involves individuals having greater self-awareness, and while respecting the needs of others, it is important that individual principles and values are not compromised (Bishop 2010).

Assertiveness links closely to communication and also self-esteem, self-efficacy and confidence that we discussed in the last chapter. If individuals are able to develop their communication skills and become more assertive, for example, saying 'no' to having sex without using a condom, then this can increase their self-esteem and self-efficacy. This can help individuals value themselves, so they feel better about themselves and can increase their belief that they can say 'no'. Having said 'no' can also lead individuals to be less critical of themselves. Assertiveness also links to problem solving, which we will discuss later in this chapter.

Getting the balance between passive assertiveness and aggressive assertiveness is not necessarily easy. Individuals may not be aware of where they are in relation to this passive–aggressive continuum.

Application to practice

Case scenario 4: David

David finds life outside prison challenging. Lack of assertiveness could contribute to these feelings.

Health promotion activities:

- Ask David to think about situations when he is at home, is homeless and in prison.

- Ask him to think about 'a) does he avoid the situation b) find it difficult to be assertive most of the time c) find it difficult some of the time or d) find it easy to be assertive?' (Bishop 2010: 36).

- What happens that makes him react in a passive or aggressive manner?

- What situations make him feel that he can be assertive?

> **Key point**
>
> Health promotion work can empower individuals to identify areas of their life where they would like to be more assertive

This will identify aspects of David's life where he could develop his assertiveness skills and thereby his confidence and self-esteem.

Assertiveness training

One of the key aims of assertiveness training is to facilitate positive thinking. Individuals who think positively and communicate in a positive manner are more likely to achieve win:win situations and are more likely to have high self-esteem and self-efficacy. Developing communication skills (verbal, non-verbal and active listening) as discussed will help individuals to feel more assertive.

> **Key point**
>
> Once David has made the behavioural intention to quit smoking and is in the contemplation stage of the Stages of Change Model then health promotion can facilitate positive thinking and communication

Application to practice

Case scenario 4: David

David has signed up for a smoking cessation group. If offered a cigarette by another prisoner, David could respond 'I really should say "no" but I can't say "no"'.

Saying 'should' is likely to increase any guilt feelings that David has about smoking and this in turn could increase his anxiety and stress levels. Using 'can't' will also add to David's feelings of low self-esteem.

Health promotion activities:

- Through discussions enable David to recognize his use of negative language.

- Practise positive thinking, for example, he could write down his thoughts in relation to his reaction when offered a cigarette, and then re-phrase these in a positive manner.

- Practise use of positive language. This could be done with the health promoter or in front of a mirror, for example, 'Thanks, I would like to have a cigarette but have made the decision not to smoke today'.

- Encourage David to practise out loud. This helps the brain to think positively.

(Bishop 2010)

Key points

Practise using positive language

Avoid using: 'I can't, I should, I'll never be able to, I'm hopeless at'

Case scenario 2: Hamed

Hamed works long hours in the family taxi business, which involves a lot of sitting; however, he does very little exercise.

Those at the support group may ask Hamed why he does not do any exercise. Hamed could respond 'I really **should** do some exercise because of my diabetes and increase in weight but I have **never been** good at sport and I **can't** say "no" to Halima's lovely meals.'

Again the words highlighted in bold are examples of negative language and negative thinking.

Health promotion activities, as suggested above would facilitate more positive thinking and use of positive language.

Assertiveness training enables individuals to be able to identify when they are being oppressed, and to be able to react in a non-aggressive, honest and open manner (Crepeau et al. 2009). By being able to express themselves more clearly, assertiveness training can empower individuals to become more autonomous with their decision making. Learning how to negotiate is another communication skill that links to assertiveness training because at times compromises may need to be agreed between the health promoter and individual, or individual and their family and/or friends (Scriven 2005). Assertiveness training therefore enables individuals to stand up for themselves. However, in order to do this they first need to recognize what assertive communication means and what skills are needed (Weiten and Lloyd 1997)

Application to practice

Case scenario 4: David

Health promotion activities:

- Work with David to identify his goals.

- Role play: David could practise using positive language with either the nurse or prison staff involved with the programmes. Then once trust is established, he would practise role playing within a small group. Individuals could take turns at taking part in the role play exercise and observing. Observers could provide constructive suggestions.

- Role play: Scenarios could be used that would involve David practising making choices, and developing his communication skills, e.g. 'I feel that I want to give up but need support'.

- Body language: David could be supported to think about his use of eye contact, facial expressions and posture, and to develop an understanding that an upright but relaxed posture is useful.

- Kitchen: David works in the prison kitchen. He could be supported to identify areas of responsibility.

- He has chosen to take part in a smoking cessation and detox programme and therefore needs to take responsibility for choices he makes. Developing problem solving skills would facilitate this.

- Positive feedback: This should be provided for David following role play activities, so that he understands he is just as important as the others in the group and that his feedback to others is valued and important. This will show David that it is okay to make mistakes and ask for help.

- David/a group of prisoners could observe role plays incorporating passive communications, aggressive communications and assertive communications. Using this safe environment, they could then discuss the differences and practise using assertive communications within the group. One person could be the antagonist and David could practise assertive communications (Weiten and Lloyd 1997).

Life skills: problem solving

Problem solving can enhance self-efficacy and self-esteem and would enable Hamed and David to feel empowered. Problem solving is not a straightforward process as it involves a number of higher level cognitive skills, so it is important that we actively engage individuals and involve them in their health-related decision making. Crepeau et al. (2009) discuss four factors:

1   **Volition**: thinking about what needs to be done;

2 **Planning**: organizing what needs to be done, thinking about different solutions, maintaining attention to the task;

3 **Purposeful action**: translating the intention into action, beginning activity, changing to use another possible solution if needed and finishing the task;

4 **Self-regulation:** reflecting on whether the task has been achieved successfully.

Application to practice

Case scenario 4: David

David has been reassured by the promise of contact with support services when he is released.

He could be supported to plan and organize a list of contacts and phone numbers that would be useful to him. Next to each phone number he could list the possible support that could be provided.

Key points

Support David to identify his goals

Support David to break down complex activities into smaller steps

Checklists can be useful

Case scenario 2: Hamed

Hamed works long hours, enjoys his food and does very little exercise. He could be supported to explore his time management and to look at the tasks that are involved in promoting the family taxi business. He could then explore each of these tasks, and think about whether they could be done differently, for example, whether some could be delegated. Hamed could then plan some exercise activities into his schedule.

Convergent and divergent thinking

According to Pendleton and Schultz-Krohn (2006) there are another two aspects to consider; first 'convergent thinking' where the individual arrives at the solution straight away and second 'divergent thinking' where the individual considers a range of possible solutions. Once a number of solutions have been thought of then the best

Table 5.2 SOLVE

Specify the problem	Through discussions enable individuals to identify the problem
Options	Work together to come up with several possible solutions (divergent thinking)
Listen to advice	Sharing viewpoints can mean that a number of solutions are explored
Vary the solution	Thinking of different options fosters flexibility
Evaluate	It is always important to reflect and think about what whether the solution worked or not, and if so, why?

Table 5.3 Application of SOLVE to David

Specify the problem	David has identified that he finds life outside the prison a great hardship, and would like to make some changes to his life when released from prison. David could be supported to list aspects of his life that he would like to change; then prioritize these aspects and then choose the first two. Trying to change all aspects is complex and likely to lead to failure.
Options	Using divergent thinking, he could begin to think of all the possible solutions; he could then list them on a piece of paper.
Listen to advice	David has joined a group in the prison that builds on respect and understanding. Working with prison staff and the group, ideas could be shared before final actions agreed.
Vary the solution	Working in groups and one-to-one activities would enable David to share his ideas but also to gain ideas from others. This would encourage him to think of a variety of solutions.
Evaluate	David could work on one of the aspects that he would like to change while in prison. This would enable him to evaluate his choices and what worked well. It is important to focus on what went well first, and then to think about other possible solutions that could be used in the future.

solution can be identified (convergent thinking). Pendleton and Schultz-Krohn (2006: 601) go on to suggest using the technique (SOLVE) (Tables 5.2 and 5.3).

Soderback (2009: 208) identifies six steps that individuals should work through in order to develop their problem solving skills. We can see that there are similarities to SOLVE:

1   Problem identification

2   Evaluate contexts in which problem occurs

3   Brainstorming

4   Identify possible solutions

5   Implement strategies and modify if needed

6   Generalize process.

Application to practice

Case scenario 2: Hamed

Hamed and Halima have been invited to join a support group at the local community centre.

1   Problem identification: We could support Hamed and Halima to identify the health–related changes they would like to make, e.g. diet and exercise.

2   Evaluate contexts: We could support Hamed to identify possible reasons why he has put on weight recently.

3   Brainstorming: Hamed and Halima have talked with the nurse together, so we can assume they are working together to resolve Hamed's health issues.

4   We could support Halima to think about the traditional cooking methods she uses, and to think about possible strategies, e.g. has she changed the menus recently? How could she vary the menus? Could we

Key points

Brainstorming is not easy, so we could give an example of a strategy

It is empowering if Hamed and Halima then think of strategies themselves

provide some information on healthy eating and exercise? Does Hamed find it difficult to do any exercise? Is this linked to his weight?

5   Implement strategies: Hamed could begin with a walking exercise programme, and after a month, we could then encourage him to evaluate the effect that this has on his energy levels. Alternatively Hamed and Halima may prefer to enrol at the local gym, which provides personal training programmes.

6   Generalize process: If these strategies are working, then support could be given to Halima to consider solutions related to their diet.

Chapter summary

In this chapter we have emphasized that working in partnership with individuals who are considering health-related behavioural change is crucial to health promotion work. The aim of health promotion is to empower individuals, and they are less likely to feel empowered if we make health-related decisions and set goals *for* them. Therefore establishing a rapport and being empathetic, communicating clearly and negotiation are basic skills required for health promotion practitioners. Furthermore, in order to facilitate life skills such as assertiveness, communication and problem solving, there are a number of health promotion activities that we need to consider, and the focus should not solely be on health education, even though it has an important part to play in health promotion work. However, in order for behavioural change to be achieved, we must also consider how we can develop confidence, self-esteem, assertiveness and problem solving and literacy skills.

Key points

- Health promoters need to understand why empowerment is important.
- Practitioners need to create supportive environments that enable individuals and communities to feel empowered.
- A variety of health promotion activities have to be considered in order to facilitate the development of knowledge and skills that influence health-related decision making and behaviours.

- As well as knowledge and skills, the provision of opportunities to develop a feeling of self-control over life circumstances is significant to empowerment.

- Communication is an interactive and reciprocal process, and is a key skill for both the health promoter and the client.

- Life skills link closely to communication, self-esteem, self-efficacy and self-confidence.

Implications for practice

- It is important for you to think about individual personal, cognitive and social skills, otherwise individuals will not be able to use the information to promote and maintain their health.

- In order to empower others we need to feel empowered ourselves, and therefore we must be up to date with the evidence base of our practice and theories from health promotion.

- Health promotion is much wider than information giving, therefore we need to think about how we give information, as well as exploring activities that empower individuals to make health-related decisions.

- Reflecting on our own non-verbal and verbal communication skills, and improving these, enables us to work in partnership, and helps us to avoid being judgemental and making decisions on behalf of individuals.

End of chapter questions

1   How would you define empowerment?

2   Why is non-verbal communication important in health promotion?

3   What are the key principles of assertiveness training?

References

Bishop, S. (2010) *Develop Your Assertiveness*. London: Kogan Page.
Bond, P. (2006) Working in partnership for public health. In J. Micheson (ed.) *Expanding Nursing and Health Care Practice*. Cheltenham: Nelson Thornes.

Crepeau, E., Cohn, E. and Schell, B. (2009) *Willard and Spackman's Occupational Therapy*. Philadelphia, PA: Lippincott Williams and Wilkins.

Ewles, L. and Simnett, I. (2003) *Promoting Health: A Practical Guide*, 5th edn. Edinburgh: Baillière Tindall.

Hubley, J. and Copeman, J. (2008) *Practical Health Promotion*. Cambridge: Polity.

Knox, G. (2011) *40 Ice Breakers for Small Groups*. www.insight.typepad.co.uk (accessed 5 August 2011).

Macdowall, W., Bonell, C. and Davies, M. (2006) *Health Promotion Practice*. Maidenhead: Open University Press.

Mogford, E., Gould, L. and Devoght, A. (2010) Teaching critical health literacy in the US as a means to action on the social determinants of health. *Health Promotion International*, 26 (1): 4–13.

Mullins, L.J. (2010) *Management and Organisational Behaviour*. London: Pearson.

Nutbeam, D. (2000) Health literacy as a public health goal: a challenge for contemporary health education and communication strategies into the 21st century. *Health Promotion International*, 15 (3): 259–67.

Payne, M. (2000) *Teamwork in Mulitiprofessional Care*. Basingstoke: Palgrave.

Pendelton, H. and Schultz-Krohn, W. (2006) *Occupational Therapy: Practice Skills for Physical Dysfunction*. Philadelphia, PA: Elsevier.

Scriven, A. (ed.) (2005) *Health Promotion Practice: The Contribution of Nurses and Allied Health Professionals*. Basingstoke: Palgrave Macmillan.

Scriven, A. (2010) *Promoting Health: A Practical Guide*. London: Baillière Tindall Elsevier.

Silverman, J., Kurtz, S. and Draper, J. (2005) *Skills for Communicating with Patients*, 2nd edn. Oxford: Radcliffe.

Soderback, I. (2000) *International Handbook of Occupational Therapy Interventions*. New York: Springer Science.

Thompson, N. (2007) *Power and Empowerment*. Dorset: Russell House Publishing.

Tones, K. and Green, J. (2004) *Health Promotion Planning and Strategies*. London: Sage.

Weiten, W. and Lloyd, M. (1997) *Psychology Applied to Modern Life: Adjustment in the 90s*. New York: Brooks/Cole Publishing Company.

Westbrook, D., Kennerley, H. and Kirk, J. (2008) *An Introduction to Cognitive Behavioural Therapy: Skills and Applications*. London: Sage.

Wills, J. and Earle, S. (2007) Theoretical perspectives on promoting public health. In S. Earle, C. Lloyd, M. Sidell and S. Spurr (eds) *Theory and Research in Promoting Public Health*. London: Sage and Open University Press.

WHO (World Health Organisation) (1986) *The Ottawa Charter*. http://www.who.int/hpr/NPH/docs/ottawa_charter_hp.pdf (accessed 25 November 2010)

Useful resources

British Association for Behavioural and Cognitive Psychotherapies (BABCP). *Self Help*. http://www.babcp.com/Public/Self-Help.aspx (accessed 10 August 2011).

Butler, G. and Hope, T. (2007) *Manage Your Mind: The Mental Fitness Guide*, 2nd edn. Oxford: Oxford University Press.

Powell, T. (2008) *The Mental Health Handbook*. Milton Keynes: Speechmark Publishing Ltd.

Westbrook, D., Kennerley, H. and Kirk, J. (2008) *An Introduction to Cognitive Behaviour Therapy*. London: Sage.

6

Working with Groups and Communities
Mary Gottwald and Jane Goodman-Brown

Chapter contents

Introduction

This chapter moves away from discussing specific health promotion activities that could be used to improve individual well-being, and explores how those working within health promotion can work with groups and communities. It begins by defining groups and discusses the advantages and disadvantages of working with groups. This chapter then begins to explore aspects that we need to consider when planning health promotion programmes and working with groups. The second part of this chapter concerns working with communities, so we will look at the meaning of community and the benefits and limitations of working with communities. Strengthening communities will be examined through community development and social capital and there are a number of similarities between working with groups and communities that will be discussed as the chapter proceeds. We will use the case scenarios of David, Richard and Hamed to apply the theory to practice.

Learning objectives

By the end of this chapter the reader will be better able to:

- Define groups
- Compare and contrast theories of group work
- Explain the advantages and disadvantages of group work
- Identify key aspects for consideration when setting up group health promotion programmes
- Define community
- Explore the principles of community development
- Explain the concept of social capital

Defining groups

Throughout life we are members of various groups and we may be part of an informal social group, and also part of formal organizational groups at work. Jacques and Salmon (2007) identify that the minimum number of members required for a group is two, and Hubley and Copeman (2008) suggest a number of groups that we may belong to, such as representative groups, pressure groups, faith based groups, social groups, welfare groups or cultural groups, all of which form an important part of our lives. The focus of this chapter is on how those working within health promotion can establish groups and facilitate the members of these groups to work together and support each other to become empowered to improve their health and well-being.

Handy (1999: 150) defines a group as 'any collection of people who perceive themselves to be a group'. Schein (1988) defines a group as 'any number of people who interact with one another; are psychologically aware of one another; and perceive themselves to be a group' (cited in Mullins 2010: 307). Perception would therefore seem to be common to these definitions.

Jaques and Salmon (2007: 6, original emphasis) take this definition further, by defining groups 'as *more than* a collection of people when they possess all of the following qualities to a greater or lesser degree':

1 **Collective perception** Members are aware that they are working as a group.

2 **Needs** Members believe that the group will fulfil some individual needs.

3 **Shared aims** The group identify a common shared goal.

4 **Interdependence** Individuals are both mutually dependent and supportive of each other.

5 **Social organization** There are group norms and emotional relationships within the group.

6 **Interaction** In conversations that they have, individuals influence and respond to each other.

7 **Cohesiveness** Individuals want to belong to the group and want to partici-pate in discussions and take part in activities in order to achieve the common goal.

However, Sale (2005) and Mullins (2010) simplify this by identifying that there are only three key characteristics of groups:

1 individuals being aware of each other;

2 interacting with each other; and

3 having a common purpose.

Application to practice

Case scenario 3: Richard

Richard has been referred to a cardiac rehabilitation programme. He has a number of needs related to weight control, diet, exercise, smoking and alcohol. Therefore, although the group he works within may have different needs, they will all have the common purpose of improving their health and well-being.

Case scenario 4: David

David has signed up for a smoking cessation group where all prisoners within the group share this common goal.

Individuals within the groups that Richard and David belong to will be able to work together, interact and support each other.

Group development

Tuckman's (1965) model of group development is well known, and although limited empirical research has been carried out that supports the stages, it continues to be widely used. Tuckman initially identified four stages that all groups would go through, and although groups go through each stage, no specific time frame is allocated to any one, and some groups may spend longer in one stage than others:

1   forming

2   storming

3   norming

4   performing

Tuckman and Jensen (1977) carried out a review of the literature that in the main supported their model, and it was at this point that a fifth stage was included: adjourning.

Rickards and Moger (2000) provide some critique of this model, in that groups may never reach the stage of performing, and may instead go backwards to an earlier stage.

Forming

The first stage of group development would be when a team organizes a group health promotion programme. In this stage, individuals do not know each other and therefore would look to the health promoter to organize the group and provide some structure. The health promoter would need to facilitate activities that enable the group to get to know each other, and be able to identify common goals such as stopping smoking, changing diet or improving exercise levels.

Storming

Individuals in the group are getting to know each other. However, during this stage of group development, conflict may arise. Some individuals may be more vociferous and assertive and will want the group to be run in certain ways. They may challenge how the health promoter is leading the group. Health promoters will need to work with members of the group to enable everyone to participate.

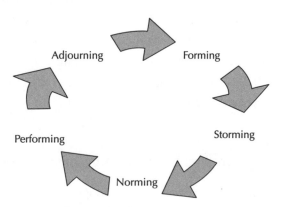

Figure 6.1 Tuckman's stages of group development

Norming

This stage is reached when the group have found ways to work together, any conflict is resolved and the group are able to cooperate and support each other. There is much greater sharing of ideas and information, and the group are able to explore options and ideas in relation to changing behaviour in order to achieve health improvement and well-being.

Performing

Mutual trust is established within the group, and members are able to work together to problem solve. The group are independent and less reliant on the health promoter as the leader.

Adjourning

Health promotion programmes may only be funded for set periods of time and therefore in this final stage the group disbands. This could be unsettling for the group members, who may have come to rely on the support provided and therefore this is a point for consideration for those who set up and led the programme. It may be useful to ensure that some follow-up contact process is established. A follow up would also identify whether the individual has relapsed and whether there is a need for inclusion in future health promotion/health improvement programmes.

For programmes that run continuously, individual members may leave the programme, either because they have achieved their goal such as stopping smoking or because they have relapsed and decided to continue with their unhealthy behaviour. While individuals may leave the programme, new members may join, and therefore the group will revert back to the 'forming' stage (adapted from Sale 2005 and Mullins 2010). Hence in Figure 6.1 Tuckman's stages of group development are seen as a cyclical process.

Groups and health promotion programmes

Scriven (2010) identifies five reasons why groups could be used with health promotion work:

144

1 raising awareness

2 mutual support

3 social action

4 education

5 group counselling.

Application to practice

Case scenario 3: Richard

As part of the cardiac rehabilitation programme Richard could join a group where **raising awareness** of the links between diet, exercise and weight are explored. Eating a healthy diet may not be the easiest choice, and living alone does not appear to motivate Richard to cook healthy meals and instead he relies on snacks. The group could provide **mutual support** by helping each other to cope with making difficult decisions, and going through difficult stages such as those experienced when taking up exercise and changing diet in order to lose weight. **Education** could be provided on the benefits of healthy eating combined with exercise and reducing alcohol intake. If members of the group have a common purpose then **group counselling** may be offered to enable them to explore the issues and possible solutions related to changing behaviour. If members of the group live in neighbourhoods where access to sports centres is limited then they could work together to campaign for social change, i.e. take **social action**. Richard has been referred to this cardiac rehabilitation programme and therefore this is likely to be time limited. At the **adjourning** stage the team will need to consider follow-up appointments and future support if needed.

Case scenario 4: David

David is part of a programme to combine health care with rehabilitation and resettlement, once released from prison. As he has signed up for a smoking cessation group, we can assume that he and other members of the group are in the contemplation stage of the Stages of Change Model (discussed in Chapter 3). In this group, the health promoter could **raise awareness** and provide **education** with the group to explore the benefits of smoking cessation and the impact of smoking on health. It could be considered cost-effective and beneficial for staff to provide **group counselling** to enable the group to share experiences of giving up smoking and different strategies that have worked previously. At the same time this would enable the group to provide **mutual support** to each other.

David will be released from prison, and has already identified that he finds life outside prison a great hardship, therefore the **adjourning** stage for him is of particular significance. He has been promised that contact with support services with be arranged on his release, so it is imperative that this is arranged otherwise David may well end up back in prison.

We discussed a variety of types of behaviour in Chapter 4, and group work could help individuals to understand their addictive behaviour and how it relates to their health so that their behaviour becomes decision based and routine behaviour. By providing mutual support, individuals may also begin to feel better about themselves and therefore their self-esteem would improve.

Therefore if groups enable individuals to work together, while at the same time taking an active part in improving their own health and well-being, we can begin to see the advantages of working in a group (Scriven 2010).

Planning health promotion programmes

Group dynamics

Table 6.1 highlights that there are both advantages and disadvantages to health promotion work when carried out in groups.

Table 6.1 Advantages and disadvantages of groups

Advantages	Disadvantages
• Provide mutual support • Raise awareness • Facilitate understanding of addictive behaviour and impact on health • Facilitate understanding of healthy behaviour and impact on health improvement • Facilitate the development of routine behaviour • Enable individuals to influence each other • Develop communication skills • Develop social skills • Develop assertiveness skills • Reduce feelings of isolation • Increase confidence • Enable sharing of knowledge • Provide opportunities for sharing experiences • Facilitate problem solving • Facilitate decision making • Trust can be established which enables members to express feelings	• Group members may be from diverse backgrounds and therefore do not have a common purpose • Health promoters may not have the skills to facilitate groups • Infrequent sessions, therefore the group do not get to know each other and move to the norming stage of group development • Members of the group keep changing and therefore it is not possible to build up trust and reach the performing stage of group development • Those who are more vociferous and assertive may dominate the group • Dominant members may not listen to others • Quieter members could feel threatened by vocal members • Members do not attend all sessions and so it is difficult to reach the performing stage of group development • Require good leadership • Require planning • Individuals have negative perceptions due to previous experience • One-to-one work may be more appropriate for some than being members of groups

Source: Hubley and Copeman (2008); Jacques and Salmon (2007); and Scriven (2010)

Activity

Think of a group that you have led.

•   What influenced your decision making, and why did you decide to run a group as opposed to working with individuals on a one-to-one basis?

•   What were the strengths of using group interventions?

- What were the limitations?

- Having explored the advantages and disadvantages above, is there anything you would do differently another time?

Therefore, when planning health promotion programmes, health promoters must think about both the advantages and disadvantages suggested above. Once these have been considered, then the decision may be made to establish a group programme or to continue to work with individuals on a one-to-one basis. It is also essential to ensure that those planning and leading the groups have the knowledge and skills to run groups and good communication skills. We discussed the importance of communication skills in Chapter 5.

Application to practice

Case scenario 3: Richard

Richard lives alone, therefore by joining a group he could benefit from talking through his concerns with others. Sharing his ideas can promote confidence, problem solving and decision making, and could lead Richard to make decisions to improve his health and well-being. Knowing that others are in a similar position with regards to health behaviours means that Richard could feel that he is not alone.

Health education activities can be included in the group work. Sharing of knowledge and strategies that have worked before can be effective in successful behavioural change.

Currently Richard tends to snack, therefore part of the group work could revolve around discussing and sharing practical tips and menus. The group could work with a dietician to plan and cook meals and also utilize opportunities to develop their cookery skills.

Although Richard says that he does not feel overly stressed, he does work long hours and has little relaxation time, therefore the health promoter could demonstrate and practise relaxation techniques with the group.

Case scenario 4: David

David has learning difficulties and a number of health-related issues linked to drug and alcohol abuse and smoking. Therefore, when selecting groups health promoters must first consider the members to avoid any bullying of David due to his learning difficulties, and second must consider the size of the group (discussed below).

By joining the smoking cessation group, David would have opportunities to share and discuss his experiences and difficulties with stopping smoking. Providing the group is not too large, he would have opportunities to develop his communication, problem solving and assertiveness skills. Development of these is likely to enhance his self-esteem and confidence.

The size of the group

The size of the group must also be considered. If the group is too small then discussions may be limited. However, if it is too big, then not everyone in the group will necessarily have an opportunity to contribute because some individuals may be more vociferous. According to Hubley and Copeman (2008), eight to

> **Key point**
>
> The size of the group can impact on the success of the group

twelve is an appropriate size but according to Handy (1999) between five and seven. Therefore when planning groups, we need to agree on the aim and purpose of the group and then consider the size.

Establishing the group

We have already discussed the strengths and limitations of group work. However, there are a number of other aspects that we need to consider when planning a health promotion programme:

- practical aspects, such as planning the venue, and timing of group sessions;

- ensuring equal access opportunities is important in relation to both the group size and venue;

- planning resources such as funding, if the venue is not hospital based. Designing and printing leaflets, arranging outside speakers and other health and social care professionals such as dieticians, physiotherapist and sports coaches;

- ensuring equal opportunities and respecting diversity are key aspects to be considered;

- at the first group meeting the group will be in Tuckman's stage of 'forming', therefore we will need to plan activities that facilitate members getting to know each other, while in a safe environment;

- making sure that the goals for each group are agreed and planned by the group, while having the support from the health promoter;

- setting and agreeing ground rules with the group members.

(adapted from Scriven 2010)

Once the group is established, the decision will need to be taken on whether the health promoter will lead the group, whether a member of the group will take on leadership responsibilities, or whether a joint partnership will be more effective (Scriven 2010). This decision is likely to arise during the 'norming and performing' stages of group development.

Impact of technology on groups

There could be an assumption that in order to build up mutual trust as identified by Scriven (2010) above, groups need to physically be together. However, when planning health promotion programmes, we ought to consider whether behavioural change could be facilitated through other means. Social media is very much part of life today, therefore we could consider whether online community groups could be established using other social media such as Facebook, Twitter, audio or video-conferencing or specific apps on iphones. Jaques and Salmon (2007) describe these as 'boundaryless groups'. If these groups are established, then the importance of setting ground rules and ensuring equal access opportunities cannot be emphasized enough.

Stop and think

- Could health promotion programmes be provided for David and Richard through the use of social media groups?
- What would be the strengths of using social media groups?
- Are there any limitations to consider?
- What influences your decision making?
- What do you need to consider when planning resources? Are there specific individual needs to think about for either David or Richard?
- How would you ensure that both David and Richard have equal access opportunities?

Health education methods

When making the decision whether to choose health promotion activities on a one-to-one basis or group basis, we should also consider how the proposed audience learns and their preferred learning style. Rogers (1969) suggests that we cannot teach but only facilitate learning, and this should underpin our planning.

Learner characteristics

The principles of adult learning remind us how adults learn (Knowles 1990):

- Adults need to feel responsible for their own learning.

- Adults have experience which should be recognized and utilized.

- Adults are more willing to learn if the learning is applicable to their coping situations.

- Adults need to see the relevance of learning.

- Motivation is internal and linked to coping with their life.

Activity choice

Activities that focus on health are most effective if they are client centred, hands on activities (Summerfield 1995, cited in Green and Tones 2010). This approach is often called active learning and includes games, simulations, role play and group work. Green and Tones (2010) suggest that selection of appropriate methods is easier if the learning objectives are precise and they are framed as behavioural objectives, for example, 'at the end of this session the learner will be able to list three strategies that could be used to stop smoking'. Links will also have to be made to ensure effective planning of health promotion programmes, otherwise behavioural objectives will not be achieved. Activity selection depends on what the learner is trying to learn. Table 6.2 highlights different methods depending on the domain. Although this is helpful in initial planning, it must be recognized that experiential learning, because of its personal nature, often encompasses more than one domain. If addressing a specific issue then learning outcomes can be tailored precisely, but if the aims are broader such as the development of empowerment, narrow outcomes will be limiting. Therefore using

> **Key point**
>
> Activity selection depends on what the learner is trying to learn

Table 6.2 Activity selection

Memorizing M	Understanding U	Doing D
Facts	Concepts Methods of learning	Skills
Association • visual • verbal Repetition • written • verbal • aura • visual Self-testing	Listening Questioning: • ourselves • others Discussing Comparing Solving problems Acting out Experiencing Imagining	Practice Demonstration Teaching others Trial and error Doing and reviewing

Source: Belbin (1981), cited in Green and Tones (2010: 316)

methods that have a multi-dimensional impact is preferable because this will allow the learner to take from a situation what they require and will lead to holistic learning (Green and Tones 2010).

Activity

- Identify a need from a programme that you are planning.

- What kind of activity do you think would be appropriate?

- What evidence supports your choice?

Stop and think

- Reflect on scenarios 3 and 4.
- Which activities would you choose to use from Table 6.2?
- What influenced your decision making?

Community

Community is very important in health promotion. We have so far focused mainly on individual health promotion; however an understanding of how health promotion can be instigated in relation to communities is essential for practice. We have already considered groups and health promotion, and there are some areas of overlap with regard to the skills you might need. Working with communities can include working with specific groups about their health issues or working on projects and campaigns, for example drugs in a children's centre or working with organizations with a wider remit than health, for instance Age UK (Scriven 2010).

This section will explore what a community is and how we encourage community involvement through participation, community development and empowerment. We will then discuss the role of social capital and apply all of these ideas to case scenario 3, Hamed.

Background

Health promotion is concerned with working with individuals and with communities. Working with communities can involve helping the community to identify their health goals, and then facilitating the achievement of these goals. Strengthening community action is one of the areas identified by the Ottawa Charter (WHO 1986) discussed in Chapter 1.

One of the major issues that is debated in relation to communities and health promotion is the definition of community, which can mean different things to different people.

Activity

- What is a community?

- How would you define a community?

Communities are often thought of as the place where people live, for example, the street or area; however a community is more complex than this, as people who live near each other may have no links or contact with each other. If we think of a street where everyone commutes to work, it may be apparent that an individual may know very little about their neighbours, and would be hard pressed to consider themselves a community.

Laverack (2004: 46) suggests a community has four components:

1   **a spatial dimension** – that is a place or locality;

2   **non-spatial dimensions** – such as interests or issues that involve people and make them a group;

3   **dynamic social relationships** – which bind people into a relationship with one another;

4   **identification of shared needs and concerns** – which can be achieved through collective action.

All four dimensions of a community need to be considered when trying to identify a given community. For example, within a geographical community there may be a number of communities that are defined by differing relationships such as gender, culture or religion. An individual can belong to a number of interest groups such as a neighbourhood improvement group or a smoking cessation group.

Application to practice

Case scenario 2: Hamed

Hamed might belong to the community that attends his local mosque (religious community); he might also belong to the Asian community within his neighbourhood (cultural community) and he might identify with both of these. He could also belong to the support group for people with diabetes at the local community centre.

Through belonging to a variety of groups and communities, individuals can take action and form a community of interest and work together to influence change (Laverack 2004). As a heath promoter we might be working with groups or communities.

Laverack's (2004) ideas help us to see that identifying a community is not as simple as it being the people who live in an area.

Activity

- Think about the communities that you belong to.

- How do they link to Laverack's (2004) four components of a community as discussed above?

There are other ways of defining communities. McMillan and Chavis (1986, cited in Tones and Tilford 2001) suggest that there are four different features of a community:

1   membership – a feeling of belonging;

2   influence – a sense of mattering;

3   integration and fulfilment of needs;

4   shared emotional connection.

This definition might alter how you perceive a community, as it is not linked to a place; it focuses on how you feel. This might be helpful if you are interested in virtual communities.

Activity

- Compare these two definitions of a community.

- Which of them is more effective in describing the communities you belong to?

Key point

Community means different things to different people

Hubley and Copeman (2008) suggest that a community can be defined in a number of ways, including a neighbourhood or an administrative unit, a social network or a group of people with similar characteristics. This range of definitions helps us to understand that defining a community is never simple. Probably the most important element in defining a community is asking the individuals involved how they perceive community and working with this definition. Therefore, as a professional working with a community it is vital to establish who is part of the community and what they want or need.

Case scenario 2: Hamed

Hamed might define his community on ethnic or religious grounds as opposed to the area in which he lives. However he might also regard the area he lives in as his community, depending on the relationship and links he has with his neighbours. McMillan and Chavis' (1986) definition of a community could be applied to Hamed. Identifying the appropriate community is important because individuals from South Asia (India, Bangladesh, Pakistan or Sri Lanka) are six times more likely to have diabetes than the rest of the UK population (NHS 2010). This situation is not found just in the UK: studies have found it to be similar in Norway and the USA (Jenum et al. 2005). This may be to do with lifestyle or it may be to do with fat storage, but improving the health of the whole community could also be appropriate. However it is important to remember that the individual must also consider diabetes to be a health issue for themselves.

Community development

While acknowledging that identifying a community is complex, it is important to be clear about who the community is in order to be able to work with it. Health promotion within communities can take place through community development but this is a contentious idea with a long history, which focuses on helping communities to identify and meet their own needs. It links to community participation, which will be discussed later.

One definition of community development is:

Community development is a way of working that encourages individual and collective action around the common needs and concerns identified by the community itself . . . it is about changing power structures to remove the barriers that prevent people from participating in the issues that affect their lives. (Standing Conference on Community Development 2006)

Community development requires three elements to be effective. It needs to be a long term process which enables people to come together, and work at their own pace. It should be based around the values of social justice, equality and respect, valuing all who are involved. Finally, its focus is on social change to address power imbalances (Community Development Exchange 2011).

This approach to health promotion emphasizes helping the community to identify their priorities and meet them through utilizing their own resources, the role of the health promoter being to help the community to help itself. Barr and Hashagen (2000) suggest that a community development approach utilizes a number of activities to help communities to increase control and develop effectiveness:

- **profiling and analysis**: helping communities to identify their strengths and areas for development;

- **capacity building**: building confidence and skills;

- **organizing**: bringing people together;

- **networking**: helping people to identify their priorities;

- **resourcing**: identifying and accessing funds;

- **negotiating**: helping the community negotiate with service providers.

> **Key point**
>
> Community capacity can be developed

Many of the ideas above are familiar to us as health promoters. However, there has been increased interest in the notion of helping a community to develop its capacity, and this has become a vital part of community development (Naidoo and Wills 2005). Developing capacity requires a community to identify its social and public health problems, and then to mobilize resources to address them. It relates to the concept of social capital which is discussed later.

Developing capacity can include identifying skills and developing them so that an individual's skills and confidence are enhanced. It can also focus on ensuring that the appropriate resources are available. If the capacity of the community is developed effectively, this will help the community to address inequalities and to move towards change. Enabling communities to develop so that they have the capacity to be healthy is one of the key components of both community development and community empowerment (Social Community Development Centre 2011).

Stop and think

- Consider Hamed's situation.
- What community abilities might need to be developed to help address the health issues?

Community development can only be successful if the members of the community participate. This in turn may lead to empowerment, so these two ideas will now be considered.

Empowerment

This concept was discussed in Chapter 5, in relation to the individual. We will now focus on empowerment in relation to communities and community development. Empowerment is a central tenet of health promotion and it is embedded in the Ottawa Charter (WHO 1986). Empowerment is about helping people to gain control over their lives both as an individual, and as a way of addressing inequalities in health. The Ottawa Charter (WHO 1986) advocates creating a supportive environment for health through building healthy public policy, and helping individuals to strengthen their own capabilities, as ways of increasing empowerment.

There are two important schools of thought about empowerment that influence health promotion:

1 Critical consciousness raising (Freire 1972).
2 Self-efficacy (Bandura 1977).

These can link to both individual and community empowerment.

Critical consciousness raising

Freire (1972) advocates liberating those who are oppressed through education, as a way of empowering them. In doing this they learn to perceive social and political contradictions, and to take action to address them. The focus is working *with* the oppressed, rather than *for* them. One aspect of this approach is that individuals are made aware that they have helped to create their culture, and so can help to transform it (Hubley and Copeman 2008). This approach to empowerment is based on a dialogue between the community and the educator, where questions are posed and answers identified in an attempt to change the situation.

Application to practice

Case scenario 2: Hamed

An example of critical consciousness raising would be that the people who attend the mosque with Hamed might be encouraged to question information about diabetes. In doing this, they could find out more about diabetes and the effects it has and the changes in lifestyle that they could adopt to help prevent it developing. This might help to empower them to change their behaviour.

Taking this approach might be more effective than telling them what to change.

Self-efficacy

Key point

Individuals and communities cannot be empowered

Bandura (1977) has a different emphasis and suggests that self-efficacy relates to an individual perception of whether they are competent in a particular situation; this approach empowers by building confidence in the individual's abilities. Bandura (1977) suggests that if an individual feels they will be able to change, then they probably will change. Therefore the emphasis is on increasing confidence.

Application to practice

Case scenario 2: Hamed

Linking this to Hamed, helping him to become empowered must focus on helping him develop his confidence, both through education and developing his practical skills. It might be that helping Hamed to develop his knowledge about food and how to cook it, could help him to feel confident to change.

Either of these approaches can be effective in helping individuals to become empowered. Tones and Tilford (2001) suggest that for self-empowerment an individual must:

- have actual power to make choices;
- believe they have control;
- have adequate life skills;

Case scenario 2: Hamed

Considering Hamed, this would mean that he could change his lifestyle through knowledge and being able to afford a change in diet, and through having the skills to change.

Therefore Tones and Tilford (2001) suggest that self-empowerment is strongly linked to personal attributes and an understanding of this is important when working with individuals. This is an important point to consider if working with Hamed, as he would need to believe that he is able to change. As health promoters, we must remember it is not possible to empower someone because empowerment links to self-belief.

Community empowerment

Community empowerment can be seen as part of the devolution of power from central government to local communities, to enable them to improve their health and well-being and reduce their need for health care services. As such it can be seen as part of the 'Big Society' advocated by the UK coalition government (DH 2010). Community empowerment is not a new idea and links to social action and involving people in their community through taking responsibility for themselves and each other.

It is suggested by Tones and Tilford (2001) that an empowered community is more than a group of empowered individuals, but it does require individuals to be empowered as they suggest that empowered individuals are more likely to participate. 'Community empowerment is both an individual and a group phenomenon . . . it is a dynamic process that never ends, involving continual shifts in individual empowerment . . . and changes in power over relations between different social groups' (Laverack 2005: 36).

This definition highlights that community empowerment is about individuals and groups working together, and is also about power. Laverack (2005) supports this idea on empowerment, in that power cannot be given but has to be gained. He suggests that there is a continuum of empowerment, from personal action to social and political action through the stages identified below:

- personal action
- development of small mutual groups
- community organizations
- partnerships
- social and political action.

Individuals begin by taking personal action, then they become involved in groups which lead to further involvement and finally social and political action.

An example might be individuals living on an estate where there is a problem with vandalism. This might impact on their mental well-being, causing them to feel stressed and anxious. A number of individuals might take action and come together to form a residents association. They may then work with other organizations such as the police and local council, leading to social action whereby vandalism is no longer tolerated by the community.

Community participation

The term 'community participation' is sometimes used instead of community development; it is also refered to as community engagement, but it is in fact a more general term and relates to the degree of involvement in a community and this links to the amount of power sharing in the community (Davies and Macdowell 2006).

One way of classifying participation and relating it to the degree of power is Arnstein's (1971) ladder (Figure 6.2). Individuals or communities can be anywhere on this continuum from non-participation to complete control.

Complete power	↑	Total control
Delegated power		Partnership
Degrees of tokenism		Placation
		Consultation
		Informing
Non-participation		Therapy
		Manipulation

Figure 6.2 Arnstein's ladder

Application to practice

Case scenario 2: Hamed

Hamed might not want to have power, or be involved in care decisions, in relation to his health issues. However, it is important that both he as an individual has the choice to be involved, and the community as a whole has choices too.

- **Non-participation** would be if the community was told what to do in relation to health, and was given no choices about the areas that were focused on.

- **Tokenism** would be if the community was informed that diabetes is an issue for the community and possibly consulted about what it would like to do in relation to this.

- **Delegated power** would be if the community was encouraged to work in partnership with professionals to address the issue of diabetes.

- **Total power** would be if the community identified the issue and took control over how resources were used in order to address the issue of diabetes, maybe through organizing community events.

Key point

Participation links to power

It is often assumed that the ultimate goal is power and total involvement, but for some communities this is not appropriate or what is desired, therefore participation and involvement along with devolution of power should depend on the community's needs. This might be influenced by the level of control individuals have over their lives, the amount of trust in the community and the degree of community cohesiveness. As well as external factors, such as the political, economic and socio-cultural situation in the community (Laverack and Wallerstein 2001), Davis and Macdowell (2006) suggest that the degree of participation that is necessary can be assessed by asking the following questions:

- What is the purpose of the work?

- To what extent do the community want to be involved?

- Are those who are engaged in the activities actually representing the community or furthering their own ambitions?

- What are the goals of the workers and is their style empowering?

The concept of community relates to empowerment and participation, and so these are important ideas that facilitate the development of health promotion.

Social capital

In recent years there has been a lot of discussion about the value of social capital in helping to protect against the ill effects of inequalities on health. Social capital focuses on the essential components of a society that enable the following characteristics to be developed (Putnam 1993)

- **existence of community networks** from families to larger networks;
- **civic engagement** participation in community networks;
- **local identity** a sense of solidarity and equality with other community members;
- **norms of trust** expectations of reciprocal help and support.

Recognizing and utilizing social capital is seen as a way of improving health: 'the concept of social capital has emerged as having potential to further articulate the relationship between health and its broader determinants. Social capital can be broadly described as the resources within a community that create family and social organisation' (Swann and Morgan 2002 : 4).

Therefore, social capital focuses on communities' connectedness, which is measured by the extent and quality of support offered within the community. Swann and Morgan (2002) further suggest that in populations that have high levels of material deprivation, a high level of social capital can act as a buffer and prevent ill health.

Social capital can be measured by the level of:

- social relationships and social support;
- formal and informal social networks;
- group memberships;
- community and civic engagements;
- shared norms and values;
- reciprocal activities such as childcare;
- level of trust in others.

> **Key point**
>
> Social capital is not a panacea for addressing inequalities in health

(Walker and Coulthard 2004)

Recognition of inequalities and the value of social capital are relevant to health promotion, as they can help in understanding the situation and resources available to help address the issues.

Application to practice

Case scenario 2: Hamed

Hamed belongs to a number of communities. However if we take his religious community as an example, this can demonstrate social capital. There are social relationships at the mosque and there are informal and formal networks as well as reciprocal activities. Informal activities might include men meeting regularly to discuss general community issues. Formal activities might be prayer groups facilitated by the Iman and reciprocal activities could include child care or looking after sick relatives.

There will also be shared norms and values. Taking these factors into account there is probably a high level of social capital which can be utilized to promote health. Begum (2003) suggests that faith based communities are among the most active social organizations and that faith appears to guarantee commitment from members.

Chapter summary

This chapter has explored the role of groups and group dynamics, including group structure and development, and the impact that these have when planning health promotion programmes. An example of the impact of group structure that was considered was the effect a new member joining a health promotion programme might have on group cohesiveness. Activities within groups have been considered and applied to practice using the case scenarios, and it is suggested that interventions are most effective if they are client centred, hands on activities.

We have explored what makes a community and acknowledged different definitions, and from this concluded that a community is best defined by the individuals within it. Communities have an important role in promoting health, and we have discussed participation and community development and linked these to the theory of community development and the situation in case scenario 2: Hamed. Furthermore, we have explored the concept of social capital and identified the key characteristics that need to be developed within communities.

Key points

- An understanding of group dynamics is vital when planning health promotion programmes.

- The purpose of a group must be clear and the advantages and disadvantages of group work should be considered.

- Groups can take place face-to-face or within the virtual environment.

- Defining communities is complex and requires negotiation with the community.

- Empowerment both for individuals and communities is essential in community health promotion work.

- The issue of social capital and the impact this has on health promotion must be considered.

Implications for practice

- Practitioners need to understand the role of groups within health promotion and to ensure that their use is appropriate.

- First of all practitioners need to work with groups to identify who the community is, and then work together to prioritize health promotion issues that need addressing.

End of chapter questions

1   When planning health promotion programmes, what factors influence decision making on whether to use group work or to work with individuals?

2   As a practitioner, how can you work with a community to enable them to become empowered in relation to their health needs?

References

Arnstein, S. (1971) Eight rungs on the ladder of citizen participation. In S. Cahn and B. Passett (eds) *Citizen Participation: Effecting Community Change*. New York: Prager.

Bandura, A. (1977) Self efficacy: towards a unifying theory of behaviour change. *Psychological Review*, 64 (2): 191–215.

Barr, A. and Hashagen, S. (2000) *ABCD Handbook: A Framework for Evaluating Community Development*. London: CDF Publications.

Begum, H. (2003) *Social Capital in Action: Adding up Local Connections and Networks*. London: Centre for Civil Society.

Community Development Exchange (2011) *Defining Community Development*. http://www.cdx.org.uk/community-development/defining-community-development (accessed 15 November 2011).

Davies, M. and Macdowall, W. (2006) *Health Promotion Theory*. Maidenhead: Open University Press.

Department of Health (2010) *Practical Approaches to Improving the Lives of Disabled and Older People Through Building Stronger Communities*. London: Department of Health.

Freire, P. (1972) *Pedagogy of the Oppressed*. London: Penguin.

Green, J. and Tones, K. (2010) *Health Promotion: Planning and Strategies*. London: Sage.

Handy, C. (1999) *Understanding Organisations*. London: Penguin.

Hubley, J. and Copeman, J. (2008) *Practical Health Promotion*. Cambridge: Polity.

Jaques, D. and Salmon, G. (2007) *Learning in Groups: A Handbook for Face:Face and Online Environments*. London: Routledge.

Jenum, A., Holme, I., Graff-Iverson, S. and Birkeland, K. (2005) Ethnicity and sex are strong determinants of diabetes in an urban Western society: implications for prevention. *Diabetiologica*, 48: 3435–9.

Knowles, M. S. (1990) *The Adult Learner: A Neglected Species*, 4th edn. London: Gulf.

Laverack, G. (2004) *Health Promotion Practice: Power and Empowerment*. London: Sage.

Laverack, G. (2005) *Public Health: Power, Empowerment and Professional Practice*. London: Sage.

Laverack, G. and Wallerstein, N. (2001) *Measuring Community Empowerment: A Fresh Look at Organizational Domains*. http://heapro.oxfordjournals.org/content/16/2/179 (accessed 4 November 2011).

McMillan, D. and Chowis, D. (1986) Sense of community: a definition and theory. *Journal of Community Psychology*, 14: 6–23.

Mullins, L. (2010) *Management and Organisational Behaviour*. London: Pearson.

Naidoo, J. and Wills, J. (2005) *Public Health and Health Promotion: Developing Practice*, 2nd edn. London: Baillière Tindall.

NHS (2010) *NHS Choice: South Asian Health Issues*. http://www.nhs.uk/Livewell/SouthAsianhealth/Pages/Overview.aspx (accessed 4 November 2011).

Putnam, R. (1993) The prosperous community: social capital and public life. *The American Prospect*, 4(13): 1–110.

Rogers, C. (1969) *Freedom to Learn*. Columbus, OH: Charles E. Merrill Publishing.

Sale, D. (2005) *Understanding Clinical Governance and Quality Assurance: Making it Happen*. Basingstoke: Palgrave Macmillan.

Scriven, A. (2010) *Promoting Health: A Practical Guide*. London: Baillière Tindall Elsevier.

Social Community Development Centre (2011) *Building Community Capacity*. http://www.scdc.org.uk/what/building-community-capacity/ (accessed 11 November 2011).

Standing Conference on Community Development (2006) www.Cdx.org.uk (accessed 11 November 2011).

Swann, C. and Morgan, A. (2002) *Social Capital for Health: Insights from Qualitative Research*. London: Health Development Agency.

Tones, K. and Tilford, S. (2001) *Health Promotion: Effectiveness, Efficiency and Equity*. London: Nelson Thornes.

Tuckman, B. (1965) Developmental sequence in small groups. *Psychological Bulletin*, 63: 384–99.

Tuckman, B. and Jensen, M. (1977) Stages of small-group development revisited. *Group and Organisational Studies*, 2(4): 419–27.

Walker, A. and Coulthard, M. (2004) Developing and understanding indicators of social capital. In A. Morgan and C. Swann (eds) *Social Capital For Health: Issues of Definition, Measurement, and Links to Health*. London: NHS Health Development Agency.

WHO (World Health Organisation) (1986) *Ottawa Charter for Health Promotion*. Geneva: WHO.

7

The Mass Media and Social Marketing
Mary Gottwald and Jane Goodman-Brown

Chapter contents

Introduction

In Chapter 5, we briefly touched on mass media approaches; this chapter will now examine their strengths and limitations in more depth. It will then examine how the choice of mass medium can be influenced by: the 'direct effects' model, which suggests that giving information will change behaviour; the diffusion of innovation theory; and the communication-behaviour change model. Lastly, we will explore the meaning of social marketing and why it is so important to identify the target group and use the mass media effectively.

We will use all four case scenarios to apply the theory to practice.

Learning objectives

By the end of this chapter the reader will be better able to:

- Critique mass media approaches and identify relevant approaches to their practice
- Compare and contrast the direct effects model, diffusion of innovation theory and communication-behaviour change model
- Explore the theory of social marketing
- Apply social marketing to practice

Mass media

Mass media is defined by Scriven (2010: 153) as

> Channels of communication to large numbers of people and includes television, radio, the internet, magazines and newspapers, books, displays and exhibitions. Leaflets and posters are also mass media when they are used on a stand-alone basis, as opposed to use as a learning aid in face-to-face communication with an individual or a group.

Although television, radio, the internet, newspapers, magazines, leaflets and pamphlets are key forms of mass media used today, there is some debate as to whether mass media is an effective communication strategy (Morrison and Bennett 2006). Communication is the sending and receiving of messages, yet we do not have any specific means of knowing whether messages delivered via mass media have not only been received but also understood. When utilizing the mass media large numbers can be reached but there is no means of making those communications specifically relevant to individuals, and therefore mass media has to be used with caution; it is often used as a form of social marketing rather than to empower choices (Green and Tones 2010). On the other hand mass media does influence everything we do, so it has the potential to impact on us at all levels.

If we return to the Stages of Change Model that we discussed in Chapter 3, mass media could be used to promote messages that would motivate individuals to make the decision to give up smoking, reduce their alcohol intake, take more exercise, use a condom, and so on. Individuals would thus move from the pre-contemplation to contemplation stage or from the contemplation to commitment stage of this model.

Strengths and limitations of mass media approaches

Activity

- Table 7.1 presents common mass media approaches used today.
- Make a note of further strengths and limitations of these different approaches.
- Which ones are likely to have the strongest impact?
- What affected your decision making?

Table 7.1 Mass media approaches

Media	Strengths	Limitations
Social media	Modern, fast access	Assumes individuals want to use social media
Email	Quick to disseminate internationally	Communications can be misunderstood
Internet	Can reach large audiences	Assumes everyone has access to a computer
Television	Visual and audio impact	Adverts are costly to produce
Newspaper	Broadsheets and tabloid newspapers can target different audiences	Accuracy of information
Magazines	Can have a visual impact	Target audience may not buy magazines
Radio	Varied methods used to convey information, e.g. plays and news items	Requires research, preparation and talent

Those involved in health promotion work will need to consider the strengths and limitations of using mass media approaches in health promotion programmes, some of which are outlined in Table 7.2.

Chapter 6 explored the meaning of community and community development and we will now examine three models that impact on the choice of mass media

Table 7.2 Critique of mass media approaches

Strengths	Limitations
Can influence choice	Top-down approach
Reaches large numbers of the population	Communications may not be relevant to individuals per se
Can be used to disseminate evidence-based health promotion practice	Communications may not be presented at a level that everyone can understand
Useful for the transmission of straightforward messages	
Effective as part of the overall health promotion strategy	Media may provide one-sided information
Effective if combined with other health promotion activities	Television and radio may represent unhealthy behaviours such as drinking and smoking as the norm without necessarily raising awareness of possible problems
Raises awareness	
Can provide links to other support, for example, telephone hot lines, leaflets, community health promotion activities	One-way communication and therefore immediate feedback on effectiveness is not possible
Individuals can access information as and when needed	Evidence does not support lasting behavioural change
Can be used for planned campaigns and advertising	
Can target niche markets	Not effective in conveying complex information
Campaigns can be at national, regional and local level	May not convey healthy messages, e.g. advertising unhealthy food
Can impact on social and political change	
Local individuals can be included in the production of television and radio community health improvement initiatives	Sufficient funding is required in order to make an impact
	Does not develop skills
Can promote the integrity and trustworthiness of local health promotion health improvement programmes	Does not necessarily achieve attitude change
Messages can present the advantages and dis-advantages of changing health-related behaviours	Does not empower individuals to make healthy choices

Source: Green and Tones (2010); Hubley and Copeman (2008); Naidoo and Wills (2009); Scriven (2010)

approaches that could be used when working with communities: the diffusion of innovation model, the direct effects/aerosol spray model and the communication-behaviour change model. Individuals may make the decision to change their health-related behaviour as a result of mass media advertising, or from observing friends and relatives who have successfully adopted a healthy lifestyle.

Restrictions on mass media approaches

Protecting Children from Unhealthy Food Marketing (British Heart Foundation 2008) is a report published by the British Heart Foundation that began to promote the need to change advertising regulations in the UK. Sweden and Quebec have also imposed restrictions on all advertising on children under 13 (Quebec) and under 12 (Sweden).

This report discusses issues with advertising regulations, and one of the key issues is that they apply to television and not to magazines, posters or social media. The Office of Communications (Ofcom) introduced some restrictions on advertising unhealthy foods to those under 16. However, although this may reduce the pressure on children to want to buy unhealthy foods, this regulation only applies to 'programmes where children make up twenty percent higher proportion of the audience than they do of the general population, which Ofcom describe as a viewing index of 120' (British Heart Foundation 2008: 8), and this therefore excludes early evening programmes such as the X Factor. Another example is that McDonald's are able to advertise during adult viewing periods, and children may also be allowed to watch television during what is considered adult viewing time.

In response to the UK Government White Paper *Choosing Health: Making Healthy Choices Easier* (2004, cited in British Heart Foundation 2008), the Committee of Advertising Practice (CAP) regulations code aims to ensure television adverts tell the truth and complies with the UK legal framework. Although this CAP identifies a number of regulations, it was not specifically developed to promote health, and therefore does not yet distinguish between healthy and unhealthy foods. However, there is a proposal that the UK adopts a nutrient profiling system, and this could help individuals to understand the difference between healthy and unhealthy foods. As yet, this code does not cover food packaging, the internet, social media and in-store point of sale promotions, although it does cover advertising in the cinema, leaflets, newspapers, magazine, posters and emails (British Heart Foundation 2008).

The UK Government has campaigned through the 5-a-day and Health4Life, but this paper goes further and proposes that the UK follows other countries such as Canada (Quebec) and Sweden, and introduces a 9pm watershed for all unhealthy food advertising. It is also proposed that further restrictions would need to cover all marketing strategies.

Activity

Reflect on the above proposals.

- Consider the four ethical principles of autonomy, beneficence (doing good), non-maleficence (doing no harm) and justice (equity and fairness).
- Are there any ethical issues that need to be considered?

Application to practice

Case scenario 1: Emily

If the UK adopts the nutrient profiling system, Emily's teacher and school nurse would need to ensure that Emily's mother, Karen, understands what this means, and understands the labelling on packaging. As Emily and her classmates grow up, lessons could facilitate their knowledge and understanding of labelling, to make choosing the healthier foods the easiest option.

The action plan that Emily's mother and school nurse designed could also include discussions on the possible influence of advertising outside of the watershed on Emily and her classmates, i.e. if they are allowed to watch television during periods that are considered 'adult viewing'.

Diffusion of innovation theory

If mass media approaches are used, then this model suggests that a few key people will disseminate and influence innovative ideas through mass media. Diffusion is defined as 'the process by which an innovation is communicated through certain channels over time among members of a social system' (Rogers 1983, cited in Nutbeam and Harris 2004: 26). At a simplistic level, this is about the ways that are used to communicate new ideas to communities, and if the idea is perceived by the community as being new, then it is considered an innovation.

We have already discussed how changing health-related behaviour can be challenging, and similarities can be seen to the diffusion of innovation theory, in that some individuals and groups will respond to new ideas quickly, while others will resist and take longer to make the decision to change their health behaviours. Rogers (1983) uses the system for classifying adopters seen in Table 7.3, based on the time it takes to adopt new innovative ideas.

Key point

It is important not to assume that everyone adopts new behavioural change ideas

In health promotion work, we therefore need to know and understand the community that we are working with. Individuals and communities are likely to

Table 7.3   Classification of adopters

Innovators	Are the minority 2–3 per cent of the population who are in the higher socio-economic group, who try out and adopt new ideas quickly. Although they may be regarded as capricious and may not be trusted in their decisions by the majority of the community, they may be able to influence the next group.
Early adopters	Form 10–20 per cent of the population who have a significant role within their community. They are more predisposed to change and have the means, whether personal, social or financial, to take on board innovation and therefore are more likely to have an influence on the rest of the community.
Early majority	Form 30–35 per cent of the population and are more willing to change and are also won over to the idea of the change being the right thing. However, although they are a larger percentage of the population they are not in positions that enable them to influence the **early adopters**.
Late majority	Also form 30–35 per cent of the population. They tend to be sceptics who doubt new ideas until their worth has been clearly demonstrated.
Laggards	Are a minority, in that they are from 10–20 per cent of the population and tend to be homogenous, isolated groups. This is the most cautious proportion of the population and they are obdurate in accepting change and may not adopt new ideas at all.

Source: Morrison and Bennett (2006); Naidoo and Wills (2009); Nutbeam and Harris (2004)

adopt new ideas if the changes provide clear advantages, and also link to the individual's and community's values and norms. They are less likely to adopt new ideas that are complex to understand and if the effectiveness is not evident. Time is also an issue, and more time and resources may be needed if the late majority and laggards are to be reached (Nutbeam and Harris 2004; Morrison and Bennett 2006).

> **Key point**
>
> Understanding community values and norms is imperative

Application to practice

Case scenario 1: Emily

As Emily is only 6, we would need to consider where her mother sits on the continuum of adopters.

Emily's mother, Karen, is a single parent, living in rented accommodation with Emily and her younger brother Josh. Emily is one of the heaviest children in the class and does not like to engage in physical activity. It is evident from the scenario that her mother is motivated, as she meets with the school nurse to discuss Emily's weight. However, if the teacher and nurse do not consider the personal, social and economic circumstances of this family, then the ideas suggested may not be adopted by Emily's mother, and as a consequence her children may continue to lead an inactive and unhealthy lifestyle. It is possible that Karen is of the *late majority* due to lack of resources.

Case scenario 2: Hamed

At this point we do not know whether Hamed is an innovator, early adopter or at the other end of the continuum and is a laggard. However, Nutbeam and Harris (2004) identify a number of characteristics of innovations that are linked with the likelihood that Hamed and Halima will make successful changes.

Hamed has put on quite a lot of weight recently, and it has been suggested that he and Halima join a support group at the local community centre. Hamed's wife is a traditional cook, so if a dietician is invited to join the group then they would need to consider relevant traditional cultural food sources. If Hamed, Halima and other members of the support group are being encouraged to eat more fruit and vegetables, then it must be available at a cost that they can afford, and the suggestions made must link to foods that are culturally important. If the menus suggested are complex, and if the equipment needed costly, then they are not likely to be adopted. Finally if the local media publish stories and information on the impact of healthy diets, then Hamed and his wife are more likely to adopt this behavioural change.

Case scenario 3: Richard

Again we do not know where Richard sits in the classification of adopters table above. We do know that he has hypertension and high cholesterol, and has had a coronary stent inserted, and therefore can be considered to sit within the high level of risk of coronary heart disease. As a deputy head, we could also make the assumption that Richard will understand the information he receives on the benefits of changing his health-related behaviour.

If we make the assumption that the cardiac rehabilitation programme facilitates and empowers Richard to adopt healthy behaviours, then we could ask him to disseminate his knowledge through his social networks. He could therefore be considered as an *early adopter* who could potentially influence the *early majority*, *late majority* and *laggard adopters*.

Case scenario 4: David

We could also make some assumptions when thinking about David. David has signed up for a smoking cessation group, and has also been offered places on a detox programme and a reading class. Developing his level of reading could impact on his level of understanding of mass media approaches used.

We could therefore perhaps make an assumption that David is an *early adopter*, because he is using his time in prison to engage in a number of programmes, and therefore is at least thinking about changing his health-related behaviour. At this point we do not know if he will be successful or not. If successful, and if he stays out of prison, then like Richard, he could be asked to share his knowledge and experiences with other prisoners, thus influencing the *early majority*, *late majority* and *laggard adopters*.

The direct effects/aerosol spray model

Originally this model was known as the direct effects model, which assumed that individuals were submissive. Therefore mass media approaches used had an instantaneous and direct impact, and individuals changed their health-related behaviour. It initially assumed, therefore, that there was a link between knowledge, attitudes and behaviour, so if individuals are 'injected' with relevant information this would lead to a behavioural change (Morrison and Bennett 2006). Naidoo and Wills (2009) and Green and Tones (2010) liken this to a hypodermic needle, in which mass media approaches are used to present powerful messages that reach the population at large instantaneously. If health-related behaviours are not adopted, then the needle used would be bigger, and the messages would become more authoritative and be more convincing.

However, this hypodermic needle analogy has been replaced by the aerosol spray model, 'as you spray it on the surface, some of it hits the target; most of it drifts away; and very little of it penetrates' (Mendelsohn 1968, cited in Naidoo and Wills 2009: 188).

If the mass media used to promote health is consistent and reinforced, then it is more likely to have an impact, and so it would seem that we are dependent on newspapers, radio, television and magazines and so on to promote information such as the

Key point

In order to have influence, mass media approaches must be repeated

associated risks linked to smoking and eating unhealthy diets, because at the very least, the message portrayed will reach some of the target population.

If the goal of mass media is to reach the target population, the mass media approaches using the aerosol spray model should be part of health promotion programmes, and should not be the sole means of communication. In this model, the approaches used can raise awareness for some, and if adopted, the innovators can influence the early adopters and early majority and therefore change may take place within communities. However, when we discussed the education approach in Chapter 2, we emphasized that increasing knowledge does not necessarily lead to behavioural change, which explains why mass media approaches can only be part of health promotion health improvement programmes.

Communication-behaviour change model

Although we have already discussed communication in Chapter 4, it is important to return to this concept. McGuire (1989, cited in Nutbeam and Harris 2004) developed the communication-behaviour change model, to steer mass media public education campaigns, with a view that these would have an impact on attitudinal and behavioural change.

Figure 7.1 explains the impact of the message will depend on who the message comes from, i.e. the source. The World Health Organisation and governments are likely to have a greater impact than local innovators (diffusion of innovation theory). Well known celebrities such as Jade Goody – who appeared

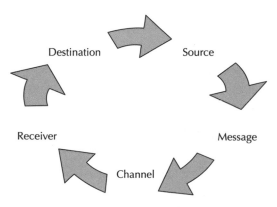

Figure 7.1 Communication-behaviour change model

on the UK television show *Big Brother* and then on the television series *Living with . . .*, and later who died from cancer – may have had more of an impact during this latter programme than unknown individuals involved in similar programmes.

This model then emphasizes that we need to think about the manner in which the message is portrayed through mass media. Television and cigarette manufacturers initially portrayed negative messages to smokers, whereas now the negative message on the impact of smoking is linked to a message providing contact numbers for help lines and smoking cessation programmes. One could question whether messages that focus on 'the benefits of not smoking' would have a bigger impact. We also should consider the medium (channel) used to deliver the message, and we have already considered the strengths and limitations of these in Table 7.1. These considerations all link to the receiver; for example, young individuals may prefer to receive a message through social media instead of going to talks and health promotion exhibitions. The last aspect of this model is the destination: has the method of communication used led to health-related behavioural change?

This model is useful in helping us to decide which medium to use when designing communication strategies for health promotion programmes. For example, when thinking about the source, it would appear that following her death from cervical cancer, the television programme Jade Goody was involved with has helped to spread the message about this preventable cancer.

Hubley and Copeman (2008) identify a number of sequences using this model that need to be well thought out in order to achieve sustained change. First of all we need to think about the target population, for example, whether they are more likely to read a broadsheet or tabloid newspaper. We need to consider the media the target population use to gain their information, as this will impact on the choices we make. Then the medium used needs first to attract attention, and then maintain it. For example, an app downloaded to an iphone may well be more attractive than a leaflet. We have already discussed the importance of understanding the message once received, however, the message also needs to be believed. If the message is believed it may lead to a change in attitude and beliefs, but it also needs to lead to behavioural change. Finally, the health improvement activities we are asking individuals to engage in must be relevant to their health concerns, otherwise successful behavioural change is less likely to take place.

Application to practice

Case scenario 4: David

Ex-prisoners or prisoners who have stopped smoking and stopped abusing drugs could be asked to produce a leaflet that identifies the benefits of changing behaviours and these could be considered an appropriate **source**. The way this **message** is portrayed is relevant, and we have already discussed the importance of language and visual impact. David is young, and therefore may well prefer to have this message delivered through **channels** that the younger generation are used to, i.e. social media. However, we must not make assumptions that social media would be his preference. These all link to the point that it is essential to consider the **receiver**. David has been reassured by the promise of contact with support services when he is released, and therefore staff can evaluate the impact on the **destination**.

Activity

Consider the four case scenarios presented in this book.

- Who is likely to be the most influential source for Emily, her mother, Hamed and Richard?

- Does the way the message is portrayed matter with each of these individuals?

- Which channels would have a greater impact in each of these case scenarios?

- How would you ensure that you consider each individual receiver?

- How could you evaluate whether the mass media communication would have impacted on the destination and successful behavioural change achieved?

- Would you include any other factors for David and if so, what influenced your decision making?

182

Table 7.4 Models that affect the choice of mass medium

Model	Disadvantages/limitations	Advantages/strengths
Diffusion of innovation theory		
The direct effects/aerosol spray model		
Communication-behaviour change model		

We have discussed three models to be considered when using mass media approaches, and the aims and advantages of these have been discussed. Reflect on these, and then consider the possible disadvantages and strengths of these models and complete Table 7.4.

Social marketing

Social marketing is the application of commercial marketing principles to health promotion in order to produce voluntary behaviour change (Grier and Bryant 2005). Basically this approach examines the needs of consumers, as well as their behaviour and attitudes towards health and their behaviour, so that health messages can be orientated specifically to the target audience and overcome some of the difficulties of using the mass media, which have already been discussed in this chapter.

Social marketing combines the knowledge of marketing principles with behaviour change theory to produce sustainable change. An example of a social marketing programme to reduce alcohol consumption is the Alcohol Effects Campaign, launched by the Department of Health in 2010. The needs of at risk drinkers are identified and the group's attitudes towards alcohol are explored. Then the programme is targeted appropriately, addressing the benefits of change, helping the target group to recognize the relevance of the campaign and examine their drinking and change their behaviour. Social marketing is not just about telling individuals what to do through using the mass media; it is an integrated campaign that supports them to change their behaviour and sustain the change in behaviour (DH 2010).

Social marketing is often used to design campaigns, and there is evidence to suggest that campaigns based on social marketing have increased impact and effectiveness (Grier and Bryant 2005). This approach to health promotion is widely used in the USA and is increasingly being used in the UK. Social marketing can be used as a planning model, and its use of behavioural theory means that it includes ideas from other models discussed earlier in the book, i.e. the importance of beliefs as discussed in the Health Belief Model and Health Action Model. Social marketing is deceptive; in this chapter it is being linked to the mass media, but it can be used more extensively and effectively to plan comprehensive interventions and campaigns (Grier and Bryant 2005).

In relation to the mass media it differs from the theories discussed above because it is based on the idea that there is a need to focus on the consumer and have an integrated approach to supporting change. Social marketing utilizes the mass media but it can also influence policy and can be about 'selling' change in behaviour too.

Social marketing has six main features, which are combined together to be effective.

1   exchange theory

2   audience segmentation

3   competition

4   marketing mix

5   consumer orientation

6   continuous monitoring

These features are explained below and linked to examples.

1 Exchange theory

This recognizes that individuals or communities are being asked to change their behaviour voluntarily, and if this is to be successful the influence of self-interest must be taken into account. This means that we need to be clear about what gives the greatest benefit at the least cost to the individual or community. The benefits are linked to a change that is of value to the individual or community. This part of social marketing theory links to the Health Belief Model, which was discussed in Chapter 3, where benefits and costs are considered and influence whether the change takes place.

184

For example, an immunization programme has to be clear about what it is that is on offer, and what the benefits to the local community are, and take account of the local situation. A campaign to promote rubella in a country where immunization is freely available and the illness is rarely seen will need to focus on different benefits from a campaign in a country where rubella occurs regularly and the immunization has to be paid for by the individual. Social marketing recognizes that the change in behaviour is voluntary, and in order to be successful the benefits need to be clearly stated.

Application to practice

Case scenario 2: Hamed

For Hamed the link to exchange theory is clear. He has to consider whether the change in diet to help control his diabetes is worth the difference it will make to his lifestyle.

The benefits of reducing the amount of fat and sugar in his diet will be that his diabetes is controlled without him having to take any medication.

The costs are that Hamed and his family will have to move away from the traditional way of cooking using ghee, and instead use lower fat alternatives. Whether or not Hamed changes will depend on how he views these costs and benefits. The role of social marketing is to help him understand the value of the change.

---

2 Audience segmentation

This recognizes that the population needs to be divided on the basis of their current behaviour, rather than on age, culture or gender. Social marketing spends a lot of time identifying who the population are, and what their current behaviour is. The more detail that is known about the targets, behaviour and attitudes, the easier it is to design an intervention to change behaviour that will be effective. The target or consumer should be at the heart of social marketing (DH 2010).

185

For example, a smoking cessation campaign aimed at teenagers who want to quit would be different to one that is designed for teenagers who don't want to stop smoking. For the first group the emphasis would be on how to stop, whereas the second group would need to have their awareness raised first. The Stages of Change Model (Prochasksa and DiClemente 1983) could be utilized here too. Social marketing recognizes that one type of intervention is not going to be effective for everyone.

Application to practice

Case scenario 1: Emily

Social marketing could help to identify what the pertinent issues are for Emily, her classmates and her family. It might be that looking at the children's behaviour at school identifies that they do not take much exercise. So the focus could be on increasing exercise as part of the school day, such as having active games at lunchtime.

Alternatively, the focus could be on Emily and her mum, recognizing that the latter might have limited cooking and shopping skills. Addressing this through community cookery classes for single mums might help Emily now, and in the future. If her mum learns to cook, then Emily might gain those skills too.

What social marketing helps us to do is to identify who the target group are and to find out from them what the issues are.

---

3 Competition

Social marketing recognizes that there are other behavioural options that compete with the healthy option. In social marketing, it is important to be clear what the alternatives to the change in health behaviour might be, and what their benefits are. Therefore it is important that effective health promotion campaigns and messages identify the advantages and challenges that are linked to the change in behaviour. A campaign using social marketing will try to make the change appear to be the most attractive option.

For example, when trying to encourage young children to eat healthily and have five pieces of fruit or vegetables a day, it is important for success that the health promoter is aware of the benefits and challenges of not eating healthily – for example, the range of foods available, gimmicks used to encourage consumption such as free toys, fun activities, easy access to fast food – to try and understand the mind-set of the children.

Recent campaigns for 5-a-day in the UK have adopted these ideas, trying to make eating fruit and vegetables 'cool' with integrated campaigns such as 'Fit 4 Life'.

This includes a fun element to encourage children to enjoy what they eat rather than focusing on the health benefits.

(For more details see: http://www.nhs.uk/change4life/Pages/Results.aspx? scope=Change4Life&q=fun&pn=1&collection=change4life&filter=0)

Looking at the benefits of a change is important, but it is also important not to try to scare people into changing as this is not effective long term. An example of this was the AIDS iceberg campaign in 1986, which tried to scare people into changing their sexual behaviour, and although cases plateaued following the campaign, the change was not sustained. It is better to focus on the tangible benefits of change rather than scaring people into changing.

Application to practice

Case scenario 4: David

David has a number of health behaviours that he could decide to change. Social marketing could help him to identify the benefits of change, while recognizing that he does have the option to continue with his current behaviour.

4 Marketing mix: the 4 Ps

Knowledge about the principles of social marketing has increased over recent years, and many people are familiar with the concept of the marketing mix. It is sometimes viewed as a standalone way of influencing the mass media; however, to be most effective it should be combined with the other five elements of social marketing.

- **Product** This refers to the characteristics and benefits associated with desired behaviour. The product could be an immunization, which has observable benefits, or a change in behaviour such as giving up smoking. Whatever the product is, it should be designed in collaboration with the target group so that it meets their needs. This may mean adapting campaigns and interventions to be appropriate for the target group rather than relying on expert views. An example in the USA was the VERB project, which aimed to increase exercise in young people. The product was changed to emphasize the fun aspect of exercise rather than the health benefits, as this made it more acceptable (Wong et al. 2004).

- **Price**: In marketing generally the price of a product is obvious. However, in social marketing the cost varies; it might be the price of an immuniza- tion, but there could be other economic costs such as having the day off to attend for screening. Or it could so be the social cost of changing behaviour, such as smoking, in that it might be part of socializing. Another cost might be the psychological loss of a pleasure, such as stopping smoking or drinking. Or it could be the psychological costs as a result of the stress of changing an addictive behaviour. The cost should be seen from the point of view of the consumer, not from the point of view of the health promoter. Making health promoting items free does not always overcome costs; for example, in the USA teenagers mistrust free condoms as possibly being inferior but will accept them if a small fee is charged (Grier and Brant 2005).

- **Place** This is where the change will take place and might include the local clinic, surgery or community centre, in which case accessibility and acceptability must be considered.

- **Promotion** This refers to the communications used to encourage change, and is quite a small part of the overall campaign or intervention. However, the kind of communication used must be appropriate to the target group. For example, young people might value communications by social media such as Facebook, but this should never be assumed. A range of communications is more effective than relying on one kind. However, these should be integrated to achieve a specific aim. For example, an intervention to increase walking to school for children would require advertising through posters and flyers, a letter to parents, skills-based sessions on road safety for the children and information sessions for parents. Decisions about what to include should be made in conjunction with the target group.

Application to practice

Case scenario 2: Richard

Richard has cardiac disease, and we can assume that he would like to prevent it worsening. Social marketing could help this by identifying clearly what the 4 Ps are for Richard.

Product Richard has choices to make about his lifestyle. He might want to improve his diet, in which case it is important to establish what the issues are for him, and find out what product would help improve his diet and he would find beneficial. It might be a series of cookery lessons or it might be joining a diet group.

Price It would be important to discuss with Richard what he considers the costs of changing his diet might be. If he enjoys his current diet, this might be difficult for him, as he will lose one of his pleasures. However, if he does not enjoy the way he eats currently, but does it because of lack of time, it will be necessary to address the issue of how to eat healthily quickly. Or he might eat the way he does because of financial pressures, in which case it is important to help him identify ways to eat healthily and cheaply.

Place This is focusing on where the change could take place; this might be at home or in the community. Is he able to access help and support at appropriate times? Is the venue where a group might be held near to him? If the issue is access to fresh food, can he get to the shops easily? Or might he need to consider other ways of doing his shopping, such as internet shopping? All of these issues need to be considered.

Promotion This is about focusing on the ways that Richard's behaviour might change. It could be a series of cookery lessons, or it might be joining a diet group. Promotion would be through advertising the classes that are available, ensuring that Richard is aware of his choices and that he has information about a change in diet.

Overall the issues here are to find out what the areas are that Richard wants to focus on and to help him to achieve his aims.

5 Consumer orientation

Consumer research is used to find out what consumers need, and to identify their priorities, as well as to increase awareness of their aspirations. It should also try to identify why they might not change. Market research helps to identify the subgroups that could be targeted, for example, those with a particular social behaviour such as excessive drinking on a Saturday night. One of the aims of having a consumer orientation is to develop a relationship with the identified target group, so that their needs are met over time, not just as a short campaign.

For example, a community exercise programme may not be successful, and so the promoters should find out why it isn't working and adapt it. By listening to the consumers' ideas, change can take place and lead to a successful intervention. Social marketing is not a top-down approach to promoting health and could be considered a bottom-up approach, as the consumer is at the centre.

6 Continuous monitoring and revision

This is an ongoing process in which the evaluation of the process, and impact of the intervention is part of the planning, and continues throughout and is vital

For example, a parenting programme for young mothers needs to be continuously monitored by group discussions or questionnaires to ensure it meets the needs of both the mothers and the children, enabling the Mums to develop appropriate skills that can be sustained beyond the duration of the course. It might mean adapting what is taught if it is not meeting the Mums' and children's needs.

Summary

Social marketing comprises six tasks, which incorporate initial planning, researching the target group, developing a strategy and then pre-testing the material. This latter is important. For example, a smoking cessation campaign in Brinnington used posters to encourage people to quit, but when these posters were pre-tested the local community found them offputting because the models held the cigarettes differently to how the locals held them. As a result the posters were changed (LGID 2010) and implementation then went ahead as did monitoring and evaluating. (Read more about this at: http://www.idea.gov.uk/idk/aio/21028178).

Application to practice

Case scenario 1: Emily

A social marketing approach means focusing on what Emily and her Mum want in order to improve their health. This might be a change in diet or a change in activity levels. Social marketing involves working with the clients to find out what they want and what the costs of change might be for them.

- **Exchange theory** To begin with, we have to help them both to identify what they will be giving up, in order to implement a change. For Emily, it might be that she enjoys watching TV, and for her Mum, it might be that she enjoys the time when Emily is quietly watching TV, so the change might be encouraging Emily and her Mum to be more active. Social marketing tries to identify solutions to problems, rather than trying to sell a product (Macdowall et al. 2006.)

- **Audience segmentation** This suggests that we should focus on Emily and her Mum's current behaviour, and help them to meet their needs rather than trying to classify them by their age or gender. It might be important here to focus on the fun element of being more active. It is important to get to know them and find out what they would like perhaps through discussion or through play.

191

- **Competition** There are many other things that Emily and her Mum might want to do and recognizing this is an important part of motivating them to change.

- **Marketing mix**

  Product is not to lose weight, but to help them have a healthier, happier future.

  Price helping them understand what they are giving up, and recognizing the benefits for Emily. For example, it might be that she will have more energy.

  Place could be vital, ensuring they can access exercise facilities, for example, the local park and swimming pool.

  Promotion is the way the change is communicated. It should be appropriate for both Emily and her Mum, for example, posters could include activities and information, and should be colourful, but they are only a small part of helping them both to change.

- **Consumer orientation** is identifying their aspirations, what they want to do, and why they want to do it. It ensures that Emily and her Mum will get what they need and be fully engaged. However, they should be consulted at all stages of the design and implementation of the intervention.

- **Continuous monitoring** includes checking that the intervention is doing what it set out to do, and is meeting the needs of both Emily and her Mum. If not, the intervention needs to be changed in order to meet their needs.

Social marketing in communities

Social marketing can be used just to design campaigns as mentioned earlier, but it could also be used fully to design integrated programmes. It can be successful at an individual level, but also at a community level. For example, in 2006 people in Knowlsley worked with the Roy Castle Lung Cancer Foundation and health organizations to produce a tailored programme for the local community which was successful (LGID 2010). It is important to recognize the unique nature of each community and focus on their needs – including consumers, health and other organizations – in the design of any programme and to take a long-term view and help people to sustain change.

Critique of social marketing

Social marketing has many advantages, but it is criticized for selling health and not always recognizing that health is not a commodity that can be measured.

It has been suggested that it is victim blaming; a downstream approach to promoting health, which looks to the individual to change their behaviour.

It has also been criticized for looking at simple solutions to complex problems, and needing to take a wider social and political focus. Despite these criticisms, it is a helpful way to get to know clients, both as individuals and communities, and to build a relationship in order to support them in their voluntary behaviour change.

Chapter summary

Mass media is an important channel of communication but when deciding which medium to use we also need to think about the advantages and disadvantages of the different media. Mass media can be used to promote health-related behaviours to large populations quickly; however, it does not necessarily achieve attitudinal and behavioural change. The diffusion of innovation theory, direct effects/aerosol spray model and the communication-behaviour change model can influence the decisions we make in relation to which medium to use. The success of adopting behaviours may depend on whether individuals are an innovator or laggard; and the way the message is delivered and the sequence in which it is delivered can also impact on whether the change is successful or not.

Social marketing applies the principles used in marketing to social situations, and focuses on the issues from the perspective of the consumer. The most well known aspect of this is looking at price, product, place and promotion and although these are important, other aspects of social marketing like consumer orientation should not be ignored.

Key points

- Mass media is not a panacea as far as health promotion is concerned.

- Mass media is useful if its use is supported by relevant theory such as diffusion of innovation or the direct effects model.

- Social marketing has six key features and in order to be effective, all need to be combined.

Implications for practice

- Health promoters need to have a clear understanding of the strengths and limitations of mass media approaches.

- The range of mass media continues to develop, so as health promoters we need to consider the appropriateness of using new technology.

- Practitioners need to understand the different aspects of social marketing in order to be able to fully utilize this approach.

End of chapter questions

1   What factors influence your choice of mass media?

2   How could the communication-behaviour change model steer the development of mass media public education campaigns?

3   How might the marketing mix influence your choice of mass media?

References

British Heart Foundation (2008) *Protecting Children from Unhealthy Food Marketing*. www.sustainweb.org/pdf/Protecting-Children_Report.pdf (accessed 9 March 2012).

DH (2010) *Alcohol: Social Marketing for England*. London: NHS.

Green, J. and Tones, K. (2010) *Health Promotion: Planning and Strategies*. London: Sage.

Grier, C. and Bryant, S. (2005) Social marketing in public health. *Annual Review of Public Health*, 26(1): 319–39.

Hubley, J. and Copeman, J. (2008) *Practical Health Promotion*. Cambridge: Polity.

LGID (Local Government Improvement and Development) (2010) *Social Marketing Approach to Tobacco Control*. London: LGID.

Macdowall, W., Bonnell, C. and Davies, M. (2006) *Health Promotion Practice*. Maidenhead: Open University Press.

Morrison, V. and Bennett, P. (2006) *An Introduction to Health Psychology*. London: Prentice-Hall.

Naidoo, J. and Wills, J. (2009) *Foundations of Health Promotion*. London: Baillière Tindall.

Nutbeam, D. and Harris, E. (2004) *Theory in a Nutshell*: London: McGraw-Hill.

Prochaska, J. and DiClemente, C. (1983) Stages and process of self change of smoking; towards an integrative model of change. *Journal of Consulting and Clincal Psychology*, 51: 390–5.

Rogers, E. (1983) *Diffusion of Innovations*, 3rd edn. New York: Free Press.

Scriven, A. (2010) *Promoting Health: A Practical Guide*. London: Baillière Tindall.

Wong, F., Huhman, M., Asbury, L. et al. (2004) VERB™ – A social marketing campaign to increase physical activity among youth. *Preventing Chronic Disease*, 1(3): A10.

Appendix: Suggested Answers to Questions Posed in Chapters

Chapter 1

How does an understanding of health and its determinants impact on your practice?	Understanding that there is no universally agreed definition of health and that health is affected by individual beliefs and culture helps practitioners to be tolerant of others' views. This helps to avoid being judgemental and possibly blaming people for their unhealthy behaviour. Recognizing the range of determinants helps us to see that heath behaviour is often beyond individual control.
What is the difference between health inequality and health inequity?	Health inequalities explain patterns of health and disease whereas inequity identifies unfairness in access to health care and in opportunities for health.
What is the role of the World Health Organisation in promoting health and well-being?	The World Health Organisation identifies relevant priorities and works with international partners to reduce health inequalities and promote health equity throughout the world.

Chapter 2

How does an understanding of the definitions of health promotion help you to develop your practice?	Definitions help practitioners to understand that health promotion is a broad concept and involves much more than health education. It takes place in a variety of contexts, with a range of individuals and groups all of whom have different needs
How can the health promotion activities be influenced by the approach(es) and levels?	Identifying the approach(es) and levels will help determine the aims of the health promotion and therefore will influence the choice of activities.
How can government directives, e.g. healthy eating in schools, help you in your role as a health promoter?	Guidelines and recommendations are provided for those who work in different contexts, for example the UK Government's Healthy School's Toolkit. These help practitioners to support individuals to lead healthier lifestyles.

Chapter 3

If you were working with an individual whose family were all overweight who wanted to eat healthily and do some exercise, which model would guide your thinking and help you to choose appropriate health promotion activities?	The choice of model depends on personal preference, so you will need to consider which model guides your practice most effectively.
Having examined the strengths and limitations of the three models, does one offer more scope for use than the others?	In our opinion, the Stages of Change Model helps to establish whether someone is ready to change. The Health Belief Model helps us to understand beliefs and subsequent actions. The Health Action Model combines these aspects and identifies a number of areas for consideration.
Can you think of an occasion when motivational interviewing would have helped you to explore someone's readiness to change?	Motivational interviewing helps to explore attitudes towards change in a structured way. It enables the client to identify why they do or do not want to change, for example, an individual who is thinking about losing weight

Chapter 4

Are some types of behaviour more difficult to change than others?	Decision-based behaviour is the easiest to change but can be influenced by whether an individual wants to change and whether the behaviour is addictive. If the behaviour is part of the group norm then it implies there is more support for the individual who wants to change. Routine behaviour may initially be difficult to change because often we are not conscious of the behaviour.
What are the strengths and limitations of salutogenesis?	Although salutogenesis is complex, it recognizes the value of life experience. Salutongenesis focuses on enablement and the value of health as opposed to disease.
Why is it important to develop an individual's self-esteem, self-efficacy and self-confidence?	Low self-esteem, self-efficacy and self-confidence can impact on the likelihood of an individual successfully changing their behaviour. The higher an individual's self-esteem the more likely they are to initiate and sustain the change.

Chapter 5

How would you define empowerment?	Your experience will influence your definition but it is important to recognize that in order to achieve successful change a variety of opportunities need to be provided.
Why is non-verbal communication important in health promotion?	If the non-verbal and verbal communications do not match then the non-verbal tends to be stronger. We must also recognize cultural differences as these can impact on whether the communication is successful or not.
What are the key principles of assertiveness training?	Assertiveness is about being confident and clearly stating what you want without being aggressive. It is also important to take into account perspective.

Chapter 6

When planning health promotion programmes, what factors influence decision making on whether to use group work or to work with individuals?	First of all we need to consider the strengths, limitations and acceptability of group work, then whether or not group work is appropriate for the purpose, e.g. is it to raise awareness? Then it is important to consider practical issues such as planning, timing and resources. Finally it is imperative that we ensure equal access to both the venue and the group.
As a practitioner, how can you work with a community to enable them to become empowered in relation to their health needs?	We need to listen to the community and find out what they consider their needs are, and then we need to act as a resource, helping them to address their health needs. It is important to facilitate, rather than impose, professional viewpoints.

Chapter 7

What factors influence your choice of mass media?	The main factor is knowing who the group is; their educational level; and what we as health promoters are trying to achieve, for example, raising awareness and/or empowering individuals to make the decision to change their health-related behaviour.

How could the communication-behaviour change model steer the development of mass media public education campaigns?	This model helps us to consider what the source of the message is (who it is from), the content of the message (that it is appropriate), the most effective way to disseminate the message (the channel), who we are aiming at (who is going to receive the message) and the destination (whether behaviour change has occurred).
How might the marketing mix influence your choice of mass media?	The marketing mix (product, price, place and promotion) helps us to consider what we want to achieve in a holistic manner. This might influence the choice of mass media, because the promotion part of the 4 Ps helps you to choose the most appropriate way of communicating. Leaflets are commonly distributed but might not be suitable because although they may address the **place** and **promotion**, they may not consider the **price** and **product** in sufficient detail.

Index

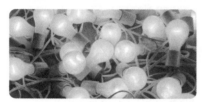
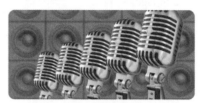
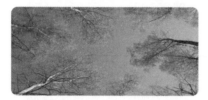
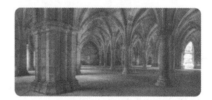
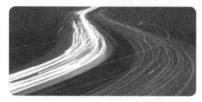
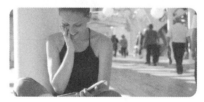
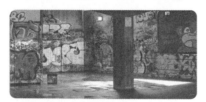

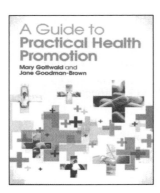

A GUIDE TO PRACTICAL HEALTH PROMOTION

Mary Gottwald and
Jane Goodman-Brown

9780335244591 (Paperback)
August 2012

eBook also available

Do you have difficulties deciding which health promotion activities facilitate behavioural change?

This accessible book focuses on the practical activity of health promotion and shows students and practitioners how to actually apply health promotion in practice. The book uses case scenarios to explore how health promotion activities can empower individuals to make decisions that change their health related behaviour

Key features:

- Each chapter uses classic case studies in health promotion
- Includes lists, key points and other succinct tools to give the reader guidance
- Contains activities and specific tasks that can be used in practice

www.openup.co.uk

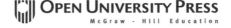

THE FUTURE PUBLIC HEALTH

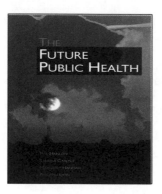

Phil Hanlon, Sandra Carlisle,
Margaret Hannah and Andrew Lyon

9780335243556 (Paperback)
February 2012

eBook also available

This innovative text bridges the gap between current public health
values and skills and those required to tackle future challenges. The
authors introduce the key models and theories of public health, as well
as the factors that have shaped its history and development.

Key features:

- Establishes the links between current public health problems and
  emerging threats like global warming and resource depletion
- Explores the true nature of modern and emerging threats to
  health
- Additional resources available from the AfterNow website
  (www.afternow.co.uk)

www.openup.co.uk

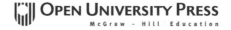

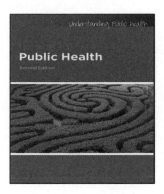

PUBLIC HISTORY AND HEALTH
Second edition

Fiona Sim and Martin McKee

9780335242641 (Paperback)
2011

eBook also available

Issues in Public Health, second edition is a text for those who want to answer the questions, 'What is public health?' and 'Why is it important?'.

This book looks at the foundations of public health, its historical evolution, the themes that underpin public health, the increasing importance of globalization and the most important causes of avoidable disease and injury. These include:

- Environmental factors
- Tobacco
- Nutrition
- Personal lifestyle factors
- Infectious disease

The second edition includes new chapters on the expanding role of public health and the impact of climate change on health. It also features expanded examples of the impact of globalization on higher and lower income countries and explores the tension between the population approach and the personal behaviour change model of health promotion.

www.openup.co.uk

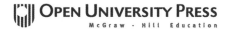

OPEN UNIVERSITY PRESS
McGraw · Hill Education